Advancing Research on Active Aging and Participation

Taina Rantanen

Advancing Research on Active Aging and Participation

A Public Health Approach

Springer

Taina Rantanen
Faculty of Sport and Health Sciences
University of Jyväskylä
Jyväskylä, Finland

ISBN 978-3-031-94701-8 ISBN 978-3-031-94702-5 (eBook)
https://doi.org/10.1007/978-3-031-94702-5

This Springer imprint is published by the registered company Springer Nature Switzerland AG
The registered company address is: Gewerbestrasse 11, 6330 Cham, Switzerland

The modern world needs people with a complex identity who are intellectually autonomous and prepared to cope with uncertainty; who are able to tolerate ambiguity and not be driven by fear into a rigid, single-solution approach to problems; who are rational and foresightful; who look for facts; who can draw inferences and can control their behavior in light of foreseen consequences, who are altruistic and enjoy doing for others; and who understand social forces and trends.

Robert J. Havighurst

Contents

Overview

1

Abstract

Traditionally, old age has been characterized as a progressive decline of health and social life. This book presents a more balanced research-based view of aging by considering older people as active agents that make decision and steer their actions to yield well-being. Considerations, concepts, theories, and research designs relevant for aging studies are discussed. Development of active aging research is followed by chapters addressing functional capacity, activities, and participation and their promotion. Old people have lived a long life, and for research of old age, the life course approach is especially pertinent. Finally, work—paid and unpaid—is explored as a form of active aging.

Long life is desired by most, and it will inevitably lead to old age. Aging of the population is one of the most significant social changes of our century. It has bearings for individuals and families, people of all ages, societal structures, consumption, education, work, transportation, housing, and cultural activities, to mention a few areas.

Old age is much more common than ever before. In fact, longevity is becoming more common than ever before in all countries. The traditional view about aging emphasized decline of health, capacity, and social life. During more recent years, a more impartial view on later life called positive gerontology redirected the focus to how older adults remain productive and engaged in meaningful roles and activities thus creating benefits to themselves and others as a result [3]. Positive gerontology will either directly or indirectly describe the benefits of engagement with life and participation in socially valued roles for personal well-being of older people. In addition, research on possibilities to promote functioning and participation are at the core of positive gerontology. However, voicing about positive aspects of old age

T. Rantanen, *Advancing Research on Active Aging and Participation*,
https://doi.org/10.1007/978-3-031-94702-5_1

is still not the mainstream in gerontology. There appears to be conceptual confusion in the field in terms of using distinct concepts.

This book aims to discuss affordances for active aging, such as environmental factors, physical and mental functioning, and literacies for different activities. These are distinct from consequences of active aging, such as well-being and quality of life that form the outcome of the process of active aging. The process of active aging at individual level in terms of individual goals, perceived abilities and opportunities, and actual activity will be discussed. Affordances for active aging are discussed from the life course perspective and from the perspective of fostering them. I suggest that active aging pertaining to individuals' goals and preferences should be defined based on the purpose of the activities rather than external criteria. For example, an important social activity "helping others" may take diverse forms, such as shoveling snow from your neighbor's yard or taking your mother to the hairdresser. Defining activities based on their purpose (such as helping) rather than providing exact external criteria for the activity (such as time use) will dissociate activities from normative assumptions concerning the operationalization of the concept of active aging [5]. Activities refer to everything that people do including physical activities, social activities, cultural activities, activities of daily life, and productive activities.

Healthy aging is a concept particularly meaningful for life course epidemiology of aging. It is often used interchangeably with active aging in studies and policy documents. However, this book views healthy aging as a concept distinct from active aging. Healthy aging refers to healthy lifestyle throughout life and reaching a high age without major health deficits. Healthy aging refers to growing old in an idealized way that is beyond reach for many people. There is an extensive body of literature about medical risks and outcomes that become increasingly common when growing old. This book will turn the attention from medical risks to a person's functioning and concentrate on abilities and activity. The concept of active aging does not take a stand on the longevity or the health status of the individual but rather on the agency of people growing old, and therefore it is inclusive and concerns everyone. Nevertheless, growing old comes with bodily changes. Muscle strength declines and mobility may become more cumbersome. These are discussed from the point of view of promoting functioning and participation and preventing disability.

The topics of this book cover research methods in aging and health and the most recent findings concerning how activity, lifestyle, and people's own actions relate to functioning, agency, and well-being in old age. It will discuss approaches to promote active aging, participation, and factors underlying it.

This book projects the recent societal changes that have made it more important than ever before to increase and disseminate knowledge about aging and old age. With increasing longevity, fewer and fewer people die before reaching old age. The onset of old age defined as the final stage of life before death cannot be precisely quantified by any biological or psychological measurements. The United Nations refers to those aged 65 years and over as old, which was also the traditional retirement age. The age limit for premature death is 70 years according to the Organisation for Economic Co-operation and Development (OECD) and the World Health

Organization (WHO). In developed countries, where life expectancy is higher, the most common age at death is around 85–90 years, and 65-year-olds may rarely be considered old. Noticeable aging changes predicting frailty and mortality become evident approximately 10 years before death, and approximately 1–3 years before death, physical and cognitive functioning start to decline more steeply [6].

With the current availability of around 20 more years of life than what the previous generations had, reconsidering life stages and social roles in more advanced ages becomes essential. The idea of 65 as a statistical threshold for old age may mislead us into thinking that life only continues from the end and that increased life expectancy merely leads to a prolongation of old age. However, life extends from the middle as well, not just the end, and old age is postponed to higher ages than before. If we consider old age to begin at the age when the expected average lifespan is around 10 years, in most developed countries, this occurs around the age of 80. However, beginning of old age is individual. It is crucial to remember that half of 80-year-olds have a life expectancy longer than 10 years, so their old age starts later. Averages depict a broad overview and not individual cases. All in all, it appears that we have a new life stage that lies approximately between the ages of 65 and 80. Members of this age group rarely perceive themselves as old; in fact, most feel younger than their age. We know that many individuals on the brink of retirement want to continue working, albeit differently. They get engaged in organizations and may contribute to care of their 90-year-old parents and young grandchildren. It appears that this age group might be a crucial pillar for the success of contemporary societies. They carry notable responsibilities for well-being of younger and older generation and for themselves.

People grow old in different historical and social circumstances. Life course studies will foster understanding about how growing old in different periods influences healthy aging; however, life course studies on active aging wait to be conducted. Increased longevity and the fact that we now have new generations of people traditionally considered as old but who do not identify as old make it imperative to look at age stages open-mindedly. This gives us in gerontology plenty of new things to study.

The roots of gerontology—the study of aging—extend far into the past, but systematic scientific research on aging became more widespread in the 1900s. The ancient Greeks suggested that as life progresses, vitality diminishes, and older people should be granted "warm baths, good food, wine, and peaceful sleep"—an active treatment approach that also today might be appreciated by many. Meanwhile, the Romans viewed old age as irreversible, but its progression could be slowed down through exercise and a suitable diet, a piece of advice that remains relevant today [4]. A significant step was the publication of scientific journals dedicated to aging research. In Europe, a German-language journal titled *Altersprobleme: Zeitschrift für Internationale Altersforschung und Altersbekämpfung* began in 1936. In the United States, the Journal of Gerontology started in 1946 and continues to be published today. In the first issue of the journal, Lawrence K. Frank wrote an article titled "Gerontologia." They emphasized the significant role gerontological research should play in determining national policies for the older people and ensuring adequate care for all those in need. They highlighted the importance of multidisciplinarity; stressed the critical reassessment of criteria for aging, especially chronological age; and proposed that diseases in old age are not necessarily normal phenomena of aging. They saw gerontology as a response to understanding and addressing the multidimensional challenges of aging, highlighting issues such as the position of aging workers, care services, technological development, and the right of people to age with dignity and equality as central themes in gerontology [2].

What will be the future of aging? People approaching old age often refer to their grandparents born in the late 1800s and form their perception of old age based on that. However, since those times, education, employment, nutrition, and healthcare have improved, and the range of possible social roles has increased. While some decades ago, it was thought that a person who had a long and strenuous career deserved to rest in old age, now older individuals want to be active and involved in the society. The ongoing positive trend in education and increased life expectancy promote a future where a growing proportion of individuals traditionally considered retirement-aged will be working. With the increasing flexibility in the working life, more and more people could work until the age of 80 or over, and the overall length of working careers may exceed 50 years. However, not all reach older ages under similar circumstances which creates disparities.

In the coming years, an increasing number of users and possibly producers of many services will be over 70 years old, and services—also other than care services—need to be increasingly directed and profiled toward the older customers due to the growing demand in this section of the population. This means that the understanding of active aging and the activities that older people prefer or need to do, and how they can best fulfill their activity needs, becomes increasingly important for the viability of various private business sectors and enterprises in addition to services provided by the public sector. To get a fresh and up-to-date idea of growing old, it is necessary to take effective measures against ageism. Ageism refers to age-based discrimination resulting from stereotypical perceptions. To alleviate ageism, older persons need to be portrayed as individuals. The media often depicts old age stereotypically with wrinkled hands and the use of walkers and slippers, creating a negative image of aging. It is important to strive for a more realistic portrayal of aging using pictures of older people going about their daily activities, such as driving a car, shopping, exercising, leading meetings, or reading newspapers.

In line with what has been the idea of gerontology since its early days, it is today characterized by the integration of various disciplines. Thus far, gerontological discovery has been greatly enriched by biomedical research approaches followed by behavioral and social sciences. Aging research seeks to promote collaboration among researchers in medicine and nursing, nutritionists, exercise and rehabilitation researchers, biologists, behavioral scientists, social scientists, social work researchers, economists, and political scientists. In fact, gerontology may be considered a magnet that attracts researchers from new disciplines [1]. The idea of this book is to look at aging from many perspectives and widen the idea of old age.

References

1. Ferraro KF. Disciplinary roots of 300 top-ranked scientific contributors to gerontology: from legacy to enriching our discovery. J Gerontol A Biol Sci Med Sci. 2022;77:2149–54.
2. Frank LK. Gerontology. J Gerontol. 1946;1:1–12.
3. Johnson KJ, Mutchler JE. The emergence of a positive gerontology: from disengagement to social involvement. The Gerontologist. 2014;54:93–100.
4. Mulley G. A history of geriatrics and gerontology. Eur Geriatr Med. 2012;3:225–7.
5. Rantanen T, Saajanaho M, Karavirta L, et al. Active aging – resilience and external support as modifiers of the disablement outcome: AGNES cohort study protocol. BMC Public Health. 2018;18:565.
6. Stolz E, Mayerl H, Muniz-Terrera G, Gill TM. Terminal decline in physical function in older adults. J Gerontol A Biol Sci Med Sci. 2024;1:79.

2 Five Considerations for Studying Active Aging and Functioning

Abstract

To get valid evidence about aging, studies should be as inclusive as possible by targeting also the oldest old section and those with disabilities. Participant involvement is paramount in studies that concern older people's well-being and services promoting well-being. To battle traditional and even ageist views about older people, it is recommended that measures assessing both positive and negative dimensions of well-being and functioning are included to create a more balanced description of the situation. Considering participant burden is a key factor in planning a successful study. It is important not to overestimate or underestimate the participants' ability to contribute. Finally, before setting up new studies, familiarizing with studies providing open-access data may be worthwhile. There may already be relevant data available which will speed up answering research question markedly.

2.1 Inclusiveness

Older people form a notable and diverse section of the existing adult population. However, they are nevertheless often excluded from studies by applying unjustified upper age limits or other criteria dismissing specific sectors of people. This results in biased information concerning populations when only people below a certain age limit are included or lack of information about older people. Such knowledge deficits may induce ageism and uninformed policies based on biased estimates and reinforce negative and stereotypic views of older people. To alleviate these risks, aging researchers need to be as inclusive as possible to involve also very old, disabled, and frail people in the studies if the idea is to gain knowledge about the general older population. However, concentrating solely in people drawn from the

T. Rantanen, *Advancing Research on Active Aging and Participation*,
https://doi.org/10.1007/978-3-031-94702-5_2

clinical context may exclude the more vigorous section of older people also biasing the view.

Missing the diversity of older people or including only measures of ill-health in studies may propel misconceptions concerning the positive as well as negative aspects of old age. For example, physical and psychological decline in old age does not necessarily exclude happiness or life satisfaction (e.g., [10]). The proportion of people in a Danish study satisfied with life remained rather stable across 10-year age groups up to 100 years even though mobility, mood, and cognitive capacity ratings decreased. Socioeconomic background is reflected in many aspects of well-being in old age. Improved functioning and self-rated health of the oldest old during past decades has been largely driven by the expansion of the higher social classes [1]. In Western countries, access to education has improved especially since the 1960s resulting in educational development. This will likely influence the socioeconomic structure of future older cohorts by increasing the proportion of those in the higher occupational classes and potentially contributing to more favorable health trajectories among older people [2]. Higher occupational class during working life and higher education mean more additional years, less multimorbidity, better functioning, and better self-rated health among the oldest old—90 years of age or older [1]. However, these positive trends do not obliterate the less favorable aging trajectories among those in high-risk, stressful jobs that exist in the society.

Oldest age groups should not be excluded from studies simply based on the assumption that they will not be able to provide appropriate and valid information. Instead, when selecting the research method, it is useful to consider that the target population may include individuals whose capacity to respond is impaired. For example, sending a mailed self-administered survey questionaire to people aged 90 years and over demonstrated that valid data may be collected this way even among the oldest old [5]. Their subsequent response rate was 81%. In this population-based study conducted in the 1990s, 71% of the home-dwelling respondents aged 90+ years lived alone, 49% went outdoors regularly, and 32% received help daily. This study was among the first to raise awareness of oldest old people living alone in the community. The other important achievement was that the authors concluded that a mailed survey was a feasible method of collecting data among the oldest old. The questionnaire consisted of 11 questions. The only open-ended question concerned the respondents' previous occupations; all others included predetermined categorizations that the respondents were asked to circle. Regardless of the brevity of the questionnaire, this study was a pathbreaker in creating knowledge about the oldest old living in the community.

It is a good idea to confirm that the interview questions are not too difficult or ambiguous to prevent confusion, fatigue, and annoyance in responding. An example of an unsuccessful attempt to collect information about well-being among older community-dwelling people comes from our own study. As part of a more extensive interview, we studied the usability of the 42-item version of the Scales of Psychological Well-being (SPWB), a widely used scale for describing self-actualization and optimal development as the foundations of well-being [8]. Our participants were 978 community-living people aged 75–85 years whose interviews were conducted by trained research assistants. The time to complete the scale ranged from 6 to 45 min, the average being 17 min. Half of the participants felt that answering the questions took a great deal of pondering. Clearly, for some participants, the burden of responding was too high, and the time it took to answer was too long. We observed that items requiring the respondent to select whether they agree or disagree with a negatively phrased statement, a two-part statement, estimation of other people's views, or comparing oneself to other people were confusing for both the respondents and the interviewers [9]. Such items should be avoided in studies among older people, possibly also in studies among people of all ages. It is important to consider that the burden of the assessments on participants is not too high.

The scales and assessments should be in line with the attributes of the study participants. Clustering of responses at the higher or lower end of the scale distribution indicates that the scale did not capture the variation as intended, and its span does not cover the characteristics of the target population. For example, basic activities of daily living (ADL) questions capture rather advanced disabilities. In a population-based community-living sample of older people, only very few will report difficulties eating, toileting, or getting dressed. Consequently, values will cluster in the end of scale describing higher performance, and data will be uninformative, unless the idea is to create a baseline for prospective study capturing new disabilities in the future. Still, development of ADL disabilities will take a long time, and such a study may not be feasible in a general population. Considering the prevalence of the condition, such as disability, in your target population will help you select a suitable assessment method that will capture variability. Disablement in old age often follows identifiable patterns of change. For declining physical capacity, the first difficulties often manifest in walking longer distances or doing other strenuous tasks such as carrying groceries up the stairs. Subsequently over time, also walking shorter distances may start to become difficult.

According to our experiences over several decades in researching physical functioning of older people, most assessments may be adapted to studies among people up to age 90 and over. Including also frail participants requires the interviews and tests to be safe and feasible for them, too. For example, individuals who have difficulty walking may not be able to take part in a long walk test, such as a 6-min test, but may be able to take part in a 10-m or a 4-m walk test, which also will provide valid information about their everyday mobility. Some people may not be able to walk at all, and for them, data on walking would be missing unless you come up with an inclusive categorization of performance. In a study by Guralnik et al. [3], the walking speed was divided into four distribution-based categories, and inability to walk was added into the variable as one category creating altogether five ascending categories: not able to walk, first (slowest), second, third, and fourth (highest) walking speed quartile. Not including in the study those unable to walk would make data less representative of the target group. In case of a physical test, not being able to carry out the assessment safely, either as perceived by the participant or the person doing the test, will likely also lead to selective drop out and bias.

2.2 Participant Involvement

Recently participant involvement in designing and conducting aging studies has received more and more attention and is now widely advocated as means to foster societal developments. In research on active aging or quality of life, for example, the people who are studied should have a say in whether the concepts are meaningful for them. Hearing the opinion of older people themselves is especially pertinent under the current circumstances when older populations are becoming increasingly diverse and their goals, needs, and preferences are changing. User involvement in research includes users as partners in different phases of the research process. Research is performed with or by users, not solely about them. The involvement of users in research enables better consideration about their needs and the acceptability of the study [4]. Thus, recruitment of participants and research quality through all stages of the research process may improve.

However, a dialogue between research participants and researchers may be problematic to conduct in equal terms. In addition, participants' views may be challenging to convert into scientifically justified research questions. In a study among aging and health researchers, the reported participant involvement most often concerned help with recruitment of study participants (43%), involving a user as a member in the advisory group (43%), providing input in the study design (40%), providing input in research questions (38%), prioritizing outcomes (35%), and identifying research topics (34%). Interpretation or disseminating results, involvement in developing the protocol, contributing to practical operations, or contributing to funding proposal were more rarely reported [6].

User involvement in aging and health studies in still not widely practiced. We have included study participants in our research in different ways. We have asked their opinions about the experience of participating in the study. This has been useful for planning the protocols for subsequent studies. More recently, we included focus group interviews in a multiphase active aging scale development process (discussed in more detail in Sect. 5.5). This was very beneficial and resulted in adding items and rephrasing some items of the scale.

2.3 Open Data

Before considering collecting new data, you may want to search whether there already exist information that are suitable and available to answer your research question. Some large studies are set up as open-ended epidemiological laboratories or infrastructures providing open-access data to researchers based on their interests. Table 2.1 lists some of the major datasets optimized for aging research that can be openly used.

These datasets are widely used in aging research and are designed to support a range of studies on health, socioeconomics, cognition, and the broader aspects of aging. Many require an application for access and compliance with data use agreements.

Table 2.1 Examples of open databases for aging research

Dataset name	Description	Data type	Access link	Notes
Health and retirement study (HRS)	A longitudinal study of health, retirement, and aging among older adults in the United States	Health, socioeconomics, cognition	hrs.isr.umich.edu	Data on U.S. adults aged 50+; includes biomarkers, interviews, and administrative records.
English longitudinal study of aging (ELSA)	Longitudinal data on the health, social, and economic circumstances of the aging population in England	Health, lifestyle, socioeconomics	ELSA Data	Tracks individuals aged 50+ over time.
Survey of health, aging and retirement in Europe (SHARE)	Multinational data on aging, health, and retirement in Europe	Health, family networks, socioeconomics	SHARE Data	Covers over 27 European countries and Israel.
National Health and aging trends study (NHATS)	US-based longitudinal study focusing on disability and aging	Health, disability, care services	NHATS Data	Tracks adults 65+ to explore trends in late-life functioning
Dementias platform UK (DPUK)	Data platform for dementia research with cohorts focusing on aging and cognition	Health, brain imaging, biomarkers	DPUK Data	Includes datasets from multiple international studies
Longitudinal aging study Amsterdam (LASA)	Research on physical, emotional, cognitive, and social functioning in the Dutch aging population	Health, social networks, cognition	LASA Data	Longitudinal data with repeated measures
Canadian longitudinal study on aging (CLSA)	Long-term study tracking health and aging among Canadians	Health, genomics, biomarkers	clsa-elv.ca	Includes 50,000 individuals aged 45–85
Global aging data repository (GADR)	Repository providing access to multiple international aging studies	Various (multi-country data)	GADR Access	Integrated platform for cross-country comparisons

National Health and Aging Trends Study (NHATS) begun in 2011in the United States; **Survey of Health, Aging and Retirement in Europe (SHARE)** was launched in 2002. **NHATS** gathers information on a nationally representative sample of Medicare beneficiaries ages 65 and older. Annual, in-person interviews collect detailed information on the disablement process and its consequences. The sample is refreshed periodically so that researchers may study national-level disability trends as well as individual trajectories. Linkages to Medicare records are also available (https://www.nhats.org/researcher/nhats, accessed 13.1.2025). **SHARE** is a research infrastructure for studying the effects of health, social, economic, and environmental policies over the life course of European citizens and beyond. In 2011 SHARE received a status in the European Research Infrastructure Consortium. SHARE is a multidisciplinary and cross-national panel database of micro data on health, socioeconomic status, and social and family networks. In seven survey waves to date, SHARE has conducted approximately 380,000 interviews with about 140,000 individuals aged 50 and over. The survey covers 28 European countries and Israel (https://share-eric.eu, accessed 13.1.2025).

2.4 Positive vs. Negative Indicators of Activity, Aging, and Health

Unlike the open-ended epidemiological aging laboratories described above, the data of researcher-led curiosity studies need to optimize data collection to specific scientifically justified questions. The measurements of the study will in the end define what questions you may answer. Traditionally the earlier landmark aging studies included measurements capturing onset of decline. As a result, positive aspects of aging did receive only limited attention. Gradually researchers have started to develop scales applicable in aging research that measure positive aspects of aging, engagement of older people in the society, and well-being. This has broadened the impression of old age and provided a more balanced view about old age. Life satisfaction, active engagement in meaningful activities, generativity, compensatory strategies, and social support are just a few examples of positive topics that have gained more attention recently.

Positive and negative aspects of aging and health are not completely exclusive and may have distinct underlying factors. This is readily understandable when considering the associations of different domains of health, i.e., psychological, social, and physical. A valid approach in studying changes when growing old should include both positive and negative aspects, and not be based on simplistic positive-only or negative-only approaches. At least, it is recommended that analyses concerning age-related changes in health and functioning should control for indicators of ill-being (such as depression or loneliness) and baseline physical health. Still today, the moderating or mediating effects of different positive psychological, behavioral, or social indicators on better health and survival are not well-known. For example, analysis of a representative sample of people living in Germany demonstrated that life satisfaction and positive affect independently predict better survival after adjustment for negative affect [11]. This finding indicates that life satisfaction and positive affect may influence survival through different, still unknown, pathways.

We studied whether the factors that increase the likelihood of high life satisfaction also decrease the likelihood of depressive symptoms among older people [7]. Depressive symptoms are more common among older than younger age groups, but life satisfaction tends to remain stable over the life course, possibly because the underlying factors or processes differ. Our research data were based on a population-based probability sample drawn from community-dwelling people aged 75, 80, and 85 years ($n = 1021$). Physical performance, perceived financial situation, executive functions, loneliness, self-acceptance, and having interests in one's life were studied as explanatory variables. The 85-year-olds, the oldest age group, reported more depressive symptoms than the 75-year-olds, the youngest age group. However, in the model including all the predictor variables age was not associated with depressive symptoms. This might indicate that having more depressive symptoms in very old age is not due to increased age but rather to lower levels of physical, social, and financial resources. The mean level of life satisfaction was similar across the three age groups. This is called "the satisfaction paradox." The ability to cope with and adapt to adversities and changes in one's life helps people to maintain an adequate level of emotional well-being, and this ability improves toward older ages. It is possible that older people adjust their reference point to what they consider is realistic in their current circumstances, a practice which may eventually fuel adaptation even in the face of losses in resources. We found that the same resources that were positively related to life satisfaction were negatively related to depressive symptoms. Our finding challenges the general idea that well-being decreases, and ill-being automatically increases with age. Instead, the diminished resources with increasing age may play a significant role in age differences. Our data did not suggest that positive and negative indicators of well-being would represent the opposite ends of one continuum. Instead, we found support for the idea that positive and negative indicators of well-being may be found in the same individual, and it is justified to include both in the same study.

2.5 Practical Issues

In the study of older individuals, specific practical challenges may arise that need to be considered in the planning. Problems may arise in the transportation of participants to the research center. In such cases, it is worth considering whether the research can be conducted at home or how transportation to the research site can be arranged. The decline in sensory abilities must be considered, for example, in the form of providing forms with a sufficiently large font size and creating quiet and undisturbed research environments. Participants may become fatigued, so preplanned rest breaks and suitable facilities should be reserved in the study center. It is a good idea to decide ahead of time what can be left unmeasured or unasked if the participants get tired. It is also necessary to be prepared to use a proxy or a substitute interviewee, such as a caregiver or family member, if the participant is no longer able to provide information. Friendly and respectful treatment is an effective way to motivate participants to complete the study.

Typically, in large studies with thousands of participants, it is necessary to find assessment methods that produce data which can relatively simply or automatically be converted into analytical files. Processing of complicated signal or structuring and categorizing open-ended questions may not be viable. In multidisciplinary studies, it is important not to overwhelm the participants with too many tests or tests perceived as too complicated. The rhythm and placement of assessments to alternate more and less demanding sections will decrease the likelihood of discontinuing. The ethical pre-evaluation needs to establish that the benefits of the research should significantly outweigh the burden and harm to the participants.

The feasibility of the planned research should be ensured, for example, through a pilot study. Gaining experience about recruiting participants and defining inclusion and exclusion criteria depending on the research purpose may bring on essential changes in the study protocol. Additionally, the required number of participants must be assessed, and for this a pilot study proves helpful. The ideal scenario is to have just the right number of participants, not too many and certainly not too few. The estimation of participant numbers is based on power calculations, which are made based on, for example, the prevalence of the phenomenon or the anticipated impact of the intervention. Throughout the research, participation activity and attrition must be monitored. The main response variables of the research must be defined before starting the study and registered in a research database maintained for this purpose. Preregistration of studies supports the researcher to cover essential planning points, while at the same time, it supports research integrity. Furthermore, the research infrastructure (measurement devices, methods, safety, communication methods, and quality system) should be carefully built and tested in advance. Ethical considerations for the research must also be assessed beforehand. Obtaining informed consent from participants is a key ethical feature. Participants must receive information about the risks associated with the research, the content of the study, the strain caused by the study, and the option to withdraw from the study if they wish. Participation must be voluntary. The recording of adverse events during the research must be planned.

References

1. Enroth L, Fors S. Trends in the social class inequalities in disability and self-rated health: repeated cross-sectional surveys from Finland and Sweden 2001-2018. Int J Public Health. 2021;66:645513.
2. Enroth L, Jasilionis D, Németh L, et al. Changes in socioeconomic differentials in old age life expectancy in four Nordic countries: the impact of educational expansion and education-specific mortality. Eur J Aging. 2022;19:161–73.
3. Guralnik JM, Simonsick EM, Ferrucci L, Glynn RJ, Berkman LF, Blazer DG, Scherr PA, Wallace RB. A short physical performance battery assessing lower extremity function: association with self-reported disability and prediction of mortality and nursing home admission. J Gerontol. 1994;2:M85–94. https://doi.org/10.1093/geronj/49.2.m85. PID: 8126356.
4. Iwarsson S, Edberg A-K, Ivanoff SD, et al. Understanding user involvement in research in aging and health. Gerontol Geriatr Med. 2019;5:2333721419897781.
5. Jylhä M, Hervonen A. Functional status and need of help among people aged 90 or over: a mailed survey with a total home-dwelling population. Scand J Public Health. 1999;2:106–11. PMID: 10421718.
6. Kylén M, Slaug B, Jonsson O, et al. User involvement in aging and health research: a survey of researchers' and older adults' perspectives. Health Res Policy Syst. 2022;20:93.

7. Pynnönen K, Kokko K, Saajanaho M, et al. Do opposite ends of same factors underlie life satisfaction vs. depressive symptoms among older people? Aging Clin Exp Res. 2021;33:2557–64.
8. Ryff CD. Happiness is everything, or is it? Explorations on the meaning of psychological wellbeing. J Pers Soc Psychol. 1989;57:1069–81.
9. Saajanaho M, Kokko K, Pynnönen K, et al. The scales of psychological wellbeing – a validation, usability and test–retest study among community-dwelling older people in Finland. Aging Ment Health. 2020;25:913–22.
10. Vestergaard S, Thinggaard M, Jeune B, et al. Physical and mental decline and yet rather happy? A study of Danes aged 45 and older. Aging Ment Health. 2015;19:400–8.
11. Wiest M, Schuz B, Webster N, et al. Subjective wellbeing and mortality revisited: differential effects of cognitive and emotional facets of wellbeing on mortality. Health Psychol. 2011;30:728–35.

Aging and Health Research Designs and Central Concepts

3

Abstract

Human studies on aging, health, and functioning are commonly categorized into observational studies and intervention studies. Observational studies aim to investigate the incidence, prevalence, and risk factors for specific outcomes and their interaction with factors like the living environment or social context, without attempting to influence these phenomena. Observational studies are often criticized for not being able to produce information on causality. Instead, observational studies will create knowledge about how common a condition is, what coincides with it, are the risks realized similarly in different environments and among different groups of people, and do some factors exacerbate or reduce the consequences of risk factors. These insights are needed when planning intervention studies. Intervention studies seek to modify the phenomenon of interest to confirm the results observed in observational studies and confirm causality. The research aim always underlies the decisions about the research design, which will be selected based on its ability to best answer the research questions posed.

3.1 Observational Studies

Cohort Study A cohort refers to people born during a specific period or to another defined group with a common characteristic. Cohort studies can be cross-sectional or longitudinal. In a cross-sectional study, people of different ages or with different characteristics related to a specific trait are studied and compared. The observed differences are interpreted as resulting from age or differences in exposures. Especially when there is little prior knowledge about the phenomenon and a foundation for further research needs to be established, cross-sectional studies are justified. The advantage is that the study is relatively quick to conduct and does not burden

T. Rantanen, *Advancing Research on Active Aging and Participation*, https://doi.org/10.1007/978-3-031-94702-5_3

participants as much as a commitment for regular follow-ups. The drawback is that temporal dynamics of the studied phenomena are not captured, and it's challenging to discern cause and effect. For example, age differences might be influenced by factors other than age, such as differences in education or past life exposures, like workplace conditions. Changes in education systems, labor laws, or healthcare principles prevailing at different times have left their mark on people's living conditions, career opportunities, and, consequently, their aging process. An example in Finland concerns 1948, when a positive and far-reaching change took place, i.e., the introduction of free school meals. It significantly improved the nutritional status of children, especially those from poorer families. The improvement in childhood nutrition positively affects health throughout the lifespan, extending to old age, and it is currently evident in increased average body height of more recently born cohorts of older people. Other important events include public health interventions, such as launching of vaccinations or new treatments.

Sequential Cohort Study Comparing people of the same age but born and living at different times provides insights into the impact on aging of societal changes or changes in living standards and lifestyles. These studies take a long time to conduct and are challenging to execute. Difficulties in interpreting results arise from standardizing research methods, the comparability of birth cohorts, and separating confounding factors from those that are part of the mechanism. For instance, improved nutrition and extended education over the decades have led to improved functional ability in the more recent generations of older individuals. Nutrition and education are underlying factors for improved functional ability. In this case, differences between birth cohorts are not necessarily derived from confounding nuisance factors but from real societal changes that have had favorable bearings on individual's health trajectories. Sequential cohort studies need to pay attention to standardizing assessment methods and recruitment procedures. Over the years, introduction of new technologies may tempt to abandon the original assessment methods, which would diminish the comparability of the past and present results.

Follow-Up Study (Prospective) Follow-up studies aim to investigate age-related changes over time in a specific cohort, the occurrence of certain diseases, or the consequences of given treatments. This type of study provides a temporal dimension, allowing us to know what happened first. It helps determine whether the assumed exposure is the cause or the consequence of the phenomenon. The advantage is the temporal aspect, and the downside is the resource-intensive nature of the study, requiring long-term commitment from researchers and participants. For the participants, the project can be burdensome. It may also be the case that the phenomenon under investigation is too rare to allow reliable modeling of its occurrence in the dataset. If the studied phenomenon is very rare, a large cohort is needed to have enough endpoint cases. This, in turn, requires too many resources and burdens a large group of participants. In follow-up studies of older individuals, the issue of selective attrition often hampers the interpretation of results. *Selective attrition* means that the sick and frail are more likely to drop out of the study than healthier individuals. In such a situation, the risk of exposures or age changes may be underestimated unless the impact of the attrition is controlled for, for example, through statistical methods and attrition analysis.

Case-Control Study When the phenomenon or disease is rare, it's justified to conduct a case-control study, searching for the causes of the disease retrospectively. A retrospective study can search, for instance, people suffering from a specific rare disease (cases) and compare them with controls who should be as similar as possible to the cases, differing only concerning the phenomenon of interest. The advantage of this research design is that it can be precisely targeted to a relatively small group of participants, gathered from various registers, requiring fewer resources, and being relatively quick to conduct. The challenge is that older people often have many diseases and functional limitations, making it difficult to define cases reliably and to find matched controls. Moreover, the studied phenomenon (disease) may have influenced assumed causes (risk factors) and led to their overestimation, i.e., the cause and the effect are reversed. An additional disadvantage is the so-called recall bias. *Recall bias* means that individuals who have experienced a certain adversity begin to search their memory for explanations for what happened in the past. In contrast, controls have not had the need to ponder this, resulting in fewer reported risk factors from their past. Recall bias causes an overestimation in exposure differences. Cognitive and memory-related problems in very old individuals may further compromise the reliability of information.

3.2 Randomized Controlled Trials (RCTs)

A randomized controlled trial (RCT) is a scientific experiment in which participants are randomly allocated to two or more groups, and each group is treated differently. RCTs require significant resources from participants, necessitating strict planning and reporting according to accepted scientific guidelines. For example, the CONSORT statement, adopted by the scientific community, is a 25-point checklist that must be followed when reporting results. An RCT should be registered before it begins. See Table 3.1 for registries. The responses of older individuals have not been extensively studied using, for example, randomized therapeutic trials because studies often select younger individuals without additional challenges. The comparison of the changes in the experimental group to the control group provides information about the benefits of the intervention. In old age, it is possible that the intervention group did not change while the control group declined. This positive effect would go unnoticed if there was not an appropriate control group.

Randomized controlled trials form the gold standard in evaluating treatment effects. Ideally, the effects ought to be relevant to the identified age groups, functional abilities, or people in specific circumstances. Interventions may be evaluated based on their external and internal validity. External validity refers to

Table 3.1 Study registries relevant for aging and health trials

Registry name	Description	Region	Website
ClinicalTrials.gov	A database of privately and publicly funded clinical studies across various health conditions, including aging-related research	Global	clinicaltrials.gov
ISRCTN Registry	A primary clinical trial registry recognized by the WHO and the ICMJE, covering aging, health, and social care studies	Global	isrctn.com
WHO International Clinical Trials Registry Platform (ICTRP)	A platform that compiles data from national and regional registries, providing access to aging-related health studies worldwide	Global	who.int/clinical-trials-registry-platform
EU Clinical Trials Register	A registry of interventional clinical trials conducted in the EU and the European Economic Area (EEA), including gerontology-related trials	Europe	clinicaltrialsregister.eu
German Clinical Trials Register (DRKS)	A national trial registry in Germany that includes studies on aging and elderly health	Germany	drks.de

generalizability or applicability of the intervention. Multiple factors underlie external validity, such as participant characteristics, intervention target, costs, compliance, and possible accompanying interventions. In practice, trials rarely can fully account for all these issues due to high costs, attrition, reduced compliance, and unexpected challenges when conducting the study. Aspects of study design, such as eligibility criteria, duration, mode and burden of the intervention, outcomes, adverse events, or statistical analysis may influence generalizability. Ensuring generalizability may compromise internal validity. Internal validity describes whether the intervention caused the observed results, and not some other factors such as chance. When study is set up so that it rules out other explanations, internal validity is high. Random allocation, allocation concealment, and blinding increase internal validity but, on the other hand, may decrease external validity. Efficacy trials aiming to determine intervention effects under ideal contexts can indicate the upper limit of benefits and have higher internal validity and possibly lower external validity. Effectiveness trials or pragmatic trials assess the benefits under "real-world" circumstances and often exhibit diluted benefits, but have higher external validity. Ideally, satisfactory internal validity accompanies generalizability.

3.3 Basic Concepts in Active Aging and Health

Age The passage of time is inevitable, and the accumulation of age is irrevocable. Old persons embody influences from their earlier life, work, social connections, and the historical period.

Chronological Age It accumulates every day, describes in a unified way how long we have lived, and is measured from birth to a given date. The year of birth gives an idea of the living conditions that prevailed during one's life. During the twentieth century, societal and technological development together with shattering historical events have left their positive and negative influences on those growing old. Chronological age forms the basis for statutory age limits, such as compulsory attendance at school, getting a driver's license, or retirement. Age of statutory majority ranges between 15 and 21 years in different countries. Age limits exist for several services. In many countries, only those above a certain age, typically 18 years, are allowed to buy alcohol. Another example concerns the higher ages. Accident insurance typically becomes unavailable for people above a certain age, often 80 years.

Even though some may wish to call chronological age merely a number, it is a highly meaningful number in gerontological research. Chronological age is the most important risk factor for many adverse outcomes, such a dementia, mobility limitations, and death.

Perceived Age People of the same chronological age can perceive their age differently. For example, most people aged 75 years do not identify with the category of "old people." Perceived age, or subjective age, reflects recognition of chronological age, societal age norms, role involvement, and health and physical limitations. Results of our earlier study among a representative sample of people aged 65–84 years showed that younger perceived age correlates with lower risk of worsening health [4]. Describing oneself as younger than one's chronological age was associated with lower risk of mortality even after adjusting for demographic factors (age, gender, educational status) and health variables (diseases, self-rated health). Of the two studied perceived age variables, perceived physical age was a stronger predictor of survival than mental age. The present data showed that participants who reported feeling "younger than their age" indeed had less diseases, a better self-rated health, a higher cognitive status score, and a lower depression score compared with people in the other perceived age categories. However, adjusting for these confounders decreased but did not eliminate its association with mortality risk. Perceived age may include more aspects than merely being an indicator of global well-being encompassing information also about factors, such as developmental expectations and cultural age norms [4]. A recent meta-analysis of 107 studies confirmed that perceived age is a robust predictor of subsequent health-related outcomes, albeit the effect is rather small [5]. Even though the number of studies on perceived age has increased over the past decade, some questions remain open. A future challenge is to explore in more detail the factors underlying the association between subjective age and future changes in health outcomes.

Social Age Social age expresses how a person behaves relative to expectations for a certain age or how mature a person is in terms of their interpersonal skills and ability to fulfill the norms and particular social roles, as compared to others of the same chronological age. Social age is derived from ratings gathered from the individual. In old age, the idea of social age leans heavily on the societal norm or expectation of behaviors associated with a certain age. For example, the age of civil majority is a key social age which varies between historical times and from one society to another. Under Roman law, girls reached their majority at age 12 and boys at age 14. In France, under the Ancien Régime, age limits for civil majority were 25 and 30, respectively. In today's world, the majority is reached between ages of 15 and 21 years depending on the country where one lives. The concept of social aging also refers to the ways in which those expectations influence what opportunities are available when growing old. One can be too young or too old for certain roles, opportunities, or benefits.

Psychological Age Psychological age describes emotional and logical maturity. In developmental psychology, stage theories contain developmental markers that most humans meet by a certain age. The developmental stages of the theories are predominantly describing childhood and young adulthood, while old age development is characterized only vaguely. For example, in Erik Erikson's stages of psychosocial development introduced in the 1950s, old age comprises a single period consisting of contemplation of life accomplishments. Stages arise as individuals grow and face new decisions and turning points during childhood, adolescence, and adulthood. As life today is much longer and social roles of older people more varied than in the 1950s when the Erikson's theory was developed, updates on psychological development in old age are called for.

Biological Age It refers to the condition and development of the body. In childhood, biological age may be defined based on genetically regulated developmental processes such as bone growth or the process of sexual maturity. In the context of aging, it can be defined as a conceptual value achieved by integrating different biomarkers of aging that assess physiological deterioration.

Cohort According to a dictionary definition, an age cohort refers to a group of people born in the same generation. In some contexts, labels may be given to people born during certain years to distinguish the lifestyles of successive generations (such as baby boomers, generation X, generation Y). The terms cohort and generation are often used interchangeably, but they are distinct concepts. Cohort refers to a group of individuals born around the same time or experiencing a certain event at the same time. Under certain conditions, a group of individuals born around the same time can become a generation, if they share more than just their birth year and develop a cultural identity for themselves. If something significant happens during the sensitive ages, such as a famine, pandemic, or war, a generational experience may be so powerful that people hold onto it even in old age. An incontestable example of shared experiences forming a generation concerns the approximately 80,000 children who were evacuated from Finland to Sweden during the Second World War to protect them from deprivation and bombings, but at the same time they were uprooted from their homes and moved into a foreign community without knowledge of the language. This is an example of generational identification having strengthened with age.

We know from empirical studies that cohorts differ from each other. For example, the perceived health of 64–69-year-olds improved from 1988 to 1996 and 2004 and were accompanied by a clear increase in the proportion of those actively engaged in physical exercise [2]. Cross-sectional studies may thus overstate age differences as those born earlier have typically lived through less propitious circumstances. Clarifying the conceptualization of age, time, and generational effects is not easy, but one can intuitively understand their existence.

Life-Course or Life Span The life course approach investigates how different exposures earlier in life influence future decisions and events, such as professional success, disease incidence, or longevity.

The five tenets of life course are time and place, life span development, timing, agency, and linked lives. Human lives are shaped by when and where they happen which makes time and place fundamental to life course research. For example, in Finland, elementary schools started to provide lunches free of charge for all pupils in the 1940s, which resulted in improved nutritional status and increased body height especially among children of poorer families, which is evident when comparing different early 1900s birth cohort to those born in the 1930s and later.

The second principle, life span development, is characterized by the view that humans develop in biologically, socially, and psychologically meaningful ways beyond childhood. Life events are not rigidly predetermined, but some abnormalities in timing (e.g. birth, growth, and development) may cause increased risk of harmful outcomes compared to those with expected timing.

Agency assumes that humans are not passive recipients of a predetermined life course but make decisions that shape their lives. Linked lives refer to social networks beyond family, such as friends, neighbors, and work associates which shape how individuals interpret life events and view prospects.

Key life course concepts include trajectory, transition, and turning point. Trajectories express the long view of life course, such as work, hobbies, or marriage. Transitions refer to passages into new life situations or roles, such as becoming a parent or grant parent or retiring from work. Transitions have a liminal quality, which means that one is not anymore here but not yet there either, a situation which may sometimes be perceived positively and sometimes negatively. Turning points involve sudden and significant change from one state to another, such as an injury or sudden onset of a disease.

Life course epidemiology is the study of long-term biological, behavioral, and psychosocial processes that link adult health and disease risk to physical or social exposures acting during gestation, childhood, adolescence, and earlier or adult life or across generations [1]. The critical period model suggests that a detrimental exposure in a critical period in life will lead to irreversible damage (e.g., mother ingesting thalidomide during pregnancy). However, early risk factors may be modified later in life as demonstrated in studies showing the increased risk of heart disease and diabetes associated with small birth weight and being further propelled by extensive childhood weight gain. Life course epidemiology is discussed in more detail in Chap. 9 of this book.

Length of Life The universal desire for longevity and the tragedy of premature death drive aging research into the topics of mortality and survival, to reveal pathways for promoting enduring and fulfilling lives. Gerontologists are intrigued by lifespan duration because, in theory, longer lives correlate with slower aging processes. Moreover, lifespan duration offers insights into public health; shorter lifespans typically coincide with a higher prevalence of diseases and injuries leading to death. Particularly in international comparisons and longitudinal studies, mortality data often stand as the most robust and comprehensive indicators of living conditions and population health [3].

Distinguishing between causes of death and predictors of mortality is crucial. Causes of death denote immediate factors leading to demise, while underlying causes initiate the fatal chain of events. In 1967, the Twentieth World Health Assembly stipulated that death certificates should include the cause of death. Causes of death encompass all diseases, pathological conditions, or injuries directly leading to or contributing to death, including the circumstances surrounding accidents or violence precipitating such injuries.

Mortality quantifies the number of deaths occurring within a population over a specified period, a fundamental metric influencing population dynamics. Alongside mortality, population change also hinges on fertility and migration. Population encompasses all inhabitants of a defined area, whether a village, municipality, state, or the entire planet. Additionally, the term "population" can extend to cohesive groups sharing common characteristics such as age, ethnicity, or language. Survival denotes the proportion of individuals who remain alive after a specified time interval following a particular event, such as reaching their 90th birthday—an inverse counterpart to mortality.

Predictors of mortality, identified years before death, indicate what factors heighten susceptibility to health decline and death. While some mortality predictors, like age and sex, remain immutable, others such as functional capacity or lifestyle choices offer avenues for modification. Epidemiological approaches enable multifaceted examinations of mortality, shedding light on biological, psychological, social, economic, and cultural influences on health and aging, thereby shaping societal mortality rates. Aging epidemiology typically concentrates on aging process indicators as mortality predictors, whereas non-communicable disease epidemiology delves into disease risk factors. Distinguishing between indicators of disease and aging processes can be challenging. Nonetheless, mortality analyses furnish insights into risk factors and conditions predisposing individuals to health decline in old age. Importantly, these risk estimates pertain to population averages and may not necessarily apply to individual contexts.

Throughout history, mortality has wielded significant influence over population growth, with population size often fluctuating in response to disease outbreaks, famines, or other catastrophic events elevating mortality rates. Even in modern times, the primary driver of global population growth has been the marked reduction in mortality rates rather than increases in fertility rates.

Person-Time Individuals may enter or exit follow-up studies at varying times. To address this variability, mortality rates are often expressed relative to person-time at risk, which combines the number of individuals with their respective time contributions in the study. Person-time represents the cumulative duration that individuals in the study population are susceptible to the conditions being investigated and serves as the primary denominator in mortality rate calculations. Only some datasets exist globally that have followed cohorts until complete extinction, with the time of death recorded for all members. However, this scenario is uncommon. More frequently, data on time to death are unavailable for all study participants, a situation termed *censoring*. Censoring occurs when information regarding the timing of an event is lacking due to loss to follow-up or the non-occurrence of the outcome event before the study's conclusion.

The hazard ratio is a key metric in epidemiology, comparing the frequency of a specific event (e.g., death) between two groups over time. It quantifies survival probabilities in an exposed group (e.g., smokers) relative to a reference group (e.g., non-smokers). A hazard ratio of one indicates no difference in survival between groups, while a value above or below one signifies increased or decreased risk, respectively. Importantly, the hazard ratio represents a relative measure of risk, rather than an absolute value.

Premature mortality, aimed at highlighting preventable deaths, is often quantified using "years of potential life lost." Premature mortality is measured in terms of potential years of life lost before a given age. World Health Organization considers deaths under 70 years of age as premature. Infant mortality, defined as death before 1 year of age, is measured by the infant mortality rate, indicating the number of infant deaths per 1000 live births.

Selective mortality is a phenomenon where individuals who are socioeconomically or otherwise disadvantaged tend to die at younger ages compared to their more advantaged counterparts. This process gradually alters the makeup of cohorts in a systematic manner, making them appear healthier, wealthier, more educated, and generally better off than they would be without this selection process. Changes in the composition of cohorts over time due to selective mortality are particularly relevant in studies involving older adults. Selective mortality leads to an underestimation of the effects being studied. Characteristics strongly associated with the risk of death may show changing prevalence over time because individuals with the highest risk are more likely to pass away, leading to a shift in the characteristics of the remaining population toward those of younger individuals.

For instance, in a study spanning 16 years, researchers found that the prevalence of poor health, as well as the proportions of men, Black individuals, unmarried individuals, and smokers declined over time when considering only those respondents who remained in the cohort in later waves. This demonstrates how selective mortality can affect the characteristics of study populations over time [6].

The landscape of risk factors is dynamic and subject to change. Advances in hygiene, public health, medicine, and nutrition over the past two centuries have significantly extended human lifespans by nearly eliminating deaths from infections. Non-communicable diseases have now become the primary causes of mortality. Looking ahead, potential cures for diseases like cancer or Alzheimer's could further alter the mortality landscape. Yet, despite ongoing increases in lifespan, there's speculation that we may be nearing the limit to human longevity. Factors such as global warming pose additional challenges, particularly for older individuals who are more vulnerable to heat waves.

The life trajectories of future cohorts of older adults will undoubtedly differ from those of current cohorts. Emerging knowledge will drive new preventive strategies and policies, potentially marginalizing certain mortality risk factors while presenting challenges for the sustainability of service systems as more people live to advanced ages.

Moreover, we're only beginning to scratch the surface of mortality studies facilitated by the aging of major cohorts established in the 1960s and beyond. As these cohorts mature, incorporating updated methodologies and conceptual frameworks, we can anticipate new insights into the mechanisms linking health risks to health decline. Advances in high-throughput biochemical and molecular analyses will provide additional data streams for investigation.

Lastly, there remain numerous factors such as biomarkers, effect modifications, interactions, additive effects, and selection biases that are yet to be fully understood, particularly within the broader older population. Additionally, individuals with specific conditions and disabilities must not be overlooked in research efforts focusing on aging and mortality. Addressing these knowledge gaps will be crucial for improving our understanding of mortality and developing effective strategies for promoting health and well-being in older populations.

References

1. Ben-Shlomo Y, Kuh D. A life course approach to chronic disease epidemiology: conceptual models, empirical challenges and interdisciplinary perspectives. Int J Epidemiol. 2002;31:285–93.
2. Heikkinen E, Kauppinen M, Rantanen T, et al. Cohort differences in health, functioning and physical activity in the young-old Finnish population. Aging Clin Exp Res. 2011;23:126–34.
3. Rantanen T. Survival, mortality and cause of death. In: Satariano WA, Maus M, editors. Aging, place and health. Burlington: Jones & Bartlett Learning; 2020. p. 69–90.
4. Uotinen V, Rantanen T, Suutama T. Perceived age as a predictor of old age mortality: a 13-year prospective study. Age Aging. 2005;34:368–72.
5. Westerhof GJ, Nehrkorn-Bailey AM, Tseng HY, et al. Longitudinal effects of subjective aging on health and longevity: an updated meta-analysis. Psychol Aging. 2023;38:147–66.
6. Zajacova A, Burgard SA. Heathier, wealthier, and wiser: a demonstration of compositional changes in aging cohorts due to selective mortality. Popul Res Policy Rev. 2013;32:311–24.

Theoretical Approaches to Aging Research

4

Abstract

Theories about aging describe, predict, and explain patterns of how people change when they grow old. They serve as frameworks for understanding complex systems and guiding further research and investigation. In scientific contexts, theories are rigorously tested and subject to scrutiny and refinement based on new evidence or insights. Early theories of aging include the disengagement theory which posits that well-being in old age stems from gradual disengagement from the society. Activity theory represents the opposing idea, i.e., active involvement in meaningful activities underlies well-being in old age. Rather than viewing aging as a problem, positive gerontology will create a more balanced view about aging. For example, with increasing age, older people may become more resilient.

The interpretation of scientific observations is closely related to the theoretical understanding of the subject in question. With theory we can explain our observations and describe what the results mean. Thus, theory is essential in the formation of new knowledge and understanding. A theory is typically based on a body of evidence, observations, experimentation, and logical reasoning. Theory does not refer to the generalizability of empirical observations. Scientific observation is generalizable when it appears in data collected from various populations, where measurements have been made validly and with reliable methods, and where there is no bias. A model describing a phenomenon, such as a model of disablement, is a structure of the connections between different levels of functioning, individual and environmental factors, and it is not a theory. Theory aims to integrate information from various observations or variables (Table 4.1). It explains how and why things are related and may also help predict the results of future scientific research. In aging

T. Rantanen, *Advancing Research on Active Aging and Participation*,
https://doi.org/10.1007/978-3-031-94702-5_4

Table 4.1 Phases of formulating a theory

Phase	Content
Observation	Observing patterns, anomalies, or questions that need explaining
Formulating questions	Asking specific questions about what underlie patterns or anomalies
Hypothesis	Formulating testable, educated guess about why or how something occurs; hypothesis need to be falsifiable so that you can prove them wrong
Experiments	Collecting appropriate data and analyzing it to provide insight about whether the hypothesis is true or not
Analyzing data	Using statistical and computational methods to assess whether data supports the hypothesis
Refinement of hypothesis	Data may support the hypothesis as is or they may require reformulating the hypothesis
Theory formulation	When several hypotheses related to a phenomenon are found to hold true, a theory explaining a broad range of observations and predicting future outcomes can be formulated
Ongoing evaluation	Theories are subjected to continuous testing and revision

research, as in other sciences, theory is a justified interpretation and explanation of observed facts. It is not the opposite of facts, and it does not stand for speculation. Aging theories aim to explain the aging process and its causes, characteristics of old age such as health, functioning, activity and well-being, consequences of aging, and how society perceives aging.

4.1 Early Theories of Aging

Early aging research was based on the idea that the prevailing feature of aging is the continuous decline in both health and social life and that old age is a problem. In 1961, Elaine Cumming and William Earl Henry introduced *the disengagement theory* [4]. The disengagement theory was the first theory of aging in the social sciences, and it created significant controversy and gave rise to more theories about older adults, their social relationships, and their societal roles. When disengagement theory emerged, there was a trend in social sciences to view that certain occurrences are necessary for the functioning of society. This idea may be echoed in one of the conjectures of the disengagement theory: the success in modern industrialized society demands certain knowledge and skill. Age-grading—where older adults retreat from their formal roles—demands that the young possess sufficient knowledge and skill to assume authority and that the old retire before they lose their skills. Either the individual, recognizing that their knowledge and skills are in decline disengages, or the organization chooses to make the individual disengage (https://www.simplypsychology.org/disengagement-theory.html, accessed 15.1.2025). According to this theory, normal aging inevitably leads to withdrawal from life roles and social disengagement, which this theory considers beneficial for the well-being of older people. An old person gradually unties from certain people or groups and social roles, spends more and more time alone, and reduces social interaction. Interaction style and, eventually, personality may change, and the persons focus more and more on themselves. This development is seen as a preparation for the ultimate disengagement, which is death. Lars Tornstam's concept of gero-transcendence, introduced in 1989, can be seen as an extension of the disengagement theory. Gero-transcendence refers to a development where an older person's perception of reality begins to change, for example, life and death are seen differently than before. A life crisis may initiate the change where the significance of casual human contacts decreases, and the importance of contemplation and the spiritual world grows, allowing the person to experience themselves in a new way. The biggest criticism against the disengagement theory and gero-transcendence is based on empirical observations showing that older adults are often forced to stand down from activities involuntarily based on negative changes in health or circumstances. This opposes disengagement theory's claim that withdrawal is voluntary and has instrumental value. Nowadays disengagement theory is largely disputed.

Activity theory began to take shape as early as the 1950s [8]. Robert J. Havighurst and Ruth Albrecht proposed that meaningful activities and engagement maintain well-being in old age. The activity theory posits that maintaining engagement in personally meaningful life situations and social interactions contribute to greater happiness, joy, and satisfaction in old age [9]. Specifically, the theory suggests that by holding on to pursuits stemming from earlier life, individuals may experience more positive life outcomes as they age [7]. Another elementary aspect of this theory is the recognition that individuals may need to substitute relinquished social roles and activities, such as those related to work, to enhance their overall well-being [9]. The loss of life content after retirement can be compensated by starting new hobbies, part-time work, or volunteering. Robert Atchley's *continuity theory*, published in the 1970s, can be seen as a further development of activity theory. With aging, individuals develop, adapt, and change in line with previous experiences and values. Yet, people strive for continuity in their values, social life, behavior, and decision-making. Continuity theory shares a similar perspective on the relationship between activity and well-being as activity theory. It posits that as individuals age, they seek to maintain their established activity patterns, which have been shaped by their preferences and abilities over their lifespan [2]. Continuity theory does not imply stagnation but advocates sustaining a degree of consistency with one's past. When individuals encounter limitations in their activities with advancing age, they may adapt to these changes by taking advantage of their accustomed knowledge, skills, and strategies. Continuity theory is best suited for interpreting situations that do not involve serious or disabling illnesses. See Table 4.2. for comparison of the social gerontological aging theories.

Table 4.2 Comparison of central tenets of social gerontological aging theories

Aspect	Disengagement theory	Activity theory	Continuity theory
Main concept	Gradual withdrawal from society is natural and beneficial	Maintaining social roles and activities leads to better well-being	Consistency in behavior and activities throughout life promotes positive aging
Role of society	Calls for disengagement as adaptation to aging	Encourages continued social involvement	Not central
Role of the individual	Accepts and adapts to withdrawal from roles	Actively seeks engagement in social and physical activities	Maintains lifestyle and behaviors and assumes new activities consistent with past patterns
Assumptions	Withdrawal is a mutual process beneficial to both society and the individual	Higher activity levels correlate with improved life satisfaction	Aging is a continuation of lifelong patterns of living
Criticisms	Ignores individual preferences and assumes withdrawal is universal. Theory discredited	Assumes high activity levels are always desired or beneficial	Limited attention to life changes that necessitate adaptation
Key proponents	Elaine Cumming, William E. Henry (1961)	Robert J. Havighurst (1960s)	Robert Atchley (1980s)
Focus areas	Social withdrawal, societal roles	Social engagement, activity	Life continuity, personal preferences
Goal	Peaceful withdrawal from societal responsibilities	Maximizing activity and engagement	Maintaining personal identity and preferences, assuming new activities to replace the old

The self-determination theory was developed by psychologists Richard Ryan and Edward Deci [5] in their book, *Intrinsic Motivation and Self-Determination in Human Behavior*. The self-determination theory was not initially directed toward aging but rather concerned children and adults in classroom or at work, but it can be relevant for regenerating aging research and research on active aging. The theory addresses motivation that underlies the best experience and best performance. Ryan and Deci present an idea of factors that facilitate or undermine motivation and discuss basic psychological needs that everybody has and that help them thrive and be motivated. The basic psychological needs that underlie activity are autonomy, competence, and relatedness. Autonomy refers to the need to make one's own decisions. Competence refers to experiencing mastery and being able to do things and produce desired outcomes. Relatedness refers to the need to feel connected with others. The criticism toward this theory is directed at its individualistic emphasis and overlook for collective motivation. The basic motivations for autonomy, competence, and relatedness will likely remain largely unchanged through most of the lifespan and spur people to take actions to fulfill these needs up to very old age even though the form of these actions may change. This theory resonates with activity theory in terms of presenting basic motivations for activity.

4.2 Positive Gerontology

Increasingly, it has been acknowledged that older individuals promote their own and others' well-being through activities in line with their goals and that they participate in society in many valuable ways. Positive gerontology opens avenues to examine aging in a more multidimensional way than what has been done before. Positive gerontology refers to research that considers aging a natural and normal part of life, and not a problem. Gerontological studies with a positive approach include measures that describe well-being, functional abilities, friendships, activity in all its forms, or life goals. By contrast, traditional gerontology has focused on studying distress, loneliness, or passivity. For example, during the last years, we have acknowledged that older people have many and diverse life goals and that they act according to their goals. Positive gerontology plays a crucial role in diversifying the image of old age within the scientific community and among the public, business, and policymakers. In this sense, positive gerontology resonates with critical gerontology originating from humanities and social sciences. Critical gerontology challenges ageist social policies and practices, such as exclusion and inequality, and promotes new retirement cultures and positive identities in later life [10].

Because traditional aging studies predominantly characterized aging as a progressive decline of health and social life, measures of ill-being, sickness, and disability have dominated studies. When researchers report the results of these measurements, they form a perception of what old age is and what growing old is like. Many positive aspects of aging may go unnoticed as such measures may not exist, or if they exist, they have not typically been included in studies. The current aging research should be challenged by conceptual analyses and by asking new questions from new perspectives to challenge the prevailing concept of old age.

Theoretical foundations are crucial because they guide the choice of variables and measurements included in the research. However, it is worth noting that there were pioneer gerontologists showing that all aging changes were not negative. Professor Erdman B. Palmore was one of the first scholars who made visible the positive aspects of aging. In his 20-year longitudinal study of persons over 60 years, he studied declines in functioning. He showed that despite the declines in health, there was little or no decline in life satisfaction or adjustment with age. The development of the skill of life satisfaction in old age is a normal part of the aging process.

4.3 Positive Aging Models

In 1997, physician John Rowe and psychologist and social scientist Robert Louis Kahn introduced the *model of successful aging*. According to this model, successful aging involves good intellectual and physical functional capacity, health, and an active lifestyle [19]. While widely known, this model has been criticized for being applicable only to a few, making it elitist. It focuses only on old age and does not consider one's previous life course. There is also criticism regarding the term "successful," as it raises the question of whether aging can be deemed unsuccessful.

Another well-known model, the *selection, optimization, and compensation (SOC) model*, created by German psychologists Paul B. Baltes and Margaret Baltes in the 1990s, emphasizes the importance of positive adaptation in successful aging. Individuals maintain their well-being and "energy balance" in old age through selection, optimization, and compensation [3]. People can compensate for the reduction in resources by adapting to their existing resources their way of doing different activities. For example, with declining physical capacities, people may walk at a slower pace or take breaks that reduce the strain on their body which enables them to continue walking and visiting destinations of interest.

The framework of active aging gained prominence in positive gerontology in the 2000s. The novelty was that the traditional view that associates the oldest stage of life with inactivity was contested. In 2002, the World Health Organization published a health policy definition of active aging. According to this definition, countries and communities should "optimize older people's opportunities for health, participation, and security to ensure the highest quality of life for them." The World Health Organization further elaborated on this concept, defining active aging as a continuous pursuit of health, participation, and security to enhance the quality of life in older age (World Health Organization 2002). This policy also emphasizes that societal measures should align with the preferences and goals of older people. See Table 4.3 for comparison of positive aging models in their central tenets. Active aging is discussed in more detail in Chap. 5 of this book.

Table 4.3 Central aspect of three positive aging models

Aspect	Successful aging model	Active aging model	Selection, optimization, and compensation (SOC) model
Main idea	Physical, cognitive, and social Well-being define successful aging	Equal opportunity to participate in activities based on personal preferences leads to good quality of life	Individuals adapt to aging by selecting goals, optimizing resources, and compensating for losses
Role of society	Not central	Should support policies promoting participation and care for those in need	Not central
Role of the individual	Proactively manages health and functioning	Engages in diverse activities for personal and social fulfillment	Actively selects priorities and finds ways to adapt to limitations. Possible for all
Criticisms	Elitistic and ignores life course. What is "unsuccessful aging?"	Policies may not pertain to individual preferences. In old age participation, e.g., in work may indicate inadequate social security	Overlooks contextual factors
Key proponents	John Rowe and Robert Kahn [19]	WHO [22]	Paul Baltes and Margret Baltes [3]
Focus areas	Health	Autonomy, participation, health, security	Goal-setting, resource management, and adaptation to changes

4.4 Resilience

Initially applied to describe the elastic properties of physical matter, resilience has since been adopted across various fields to denote the responses of systems, such as ecosystems or economies, to adverse conditions or disruptions. In the realm of human experience, resilience refers to the process of positive adaptation to or coping with life's adversities [16]. Some individuals can maintain their activity and functioning despite setbacks, while others may experience a significant decline in health and disengage from previously valued activities in similar situations. Resilience refers to the positive adaptability when facing setbacks or adversity. Exploring resilience can assist in developing interventions that promote favorable activity propelling good quality of life. In initial resilience studies, the focus was on identifying traits in children that supported positive development despite challenging circumstances. In recent years, resilience research has expanded to other age groups, including older people.

The scientific inquiry into human resilience began in the 1970s within developmental psychology, focusing on children exhibiting exceptional developmental outcomes despite early-life adversity [17]. In these studies, the resilient individuals who despite early-life adversity avoided later-life troubles, highlighted the importance of internal qualities within individuals. From these ideas, resilience research has gradually shifted toward emphasizing the intricate interplay between individuals and their environments. Resilience is now viewed as a comprehensive interaction process involving the individual, their past experiences, and their environment, rather than just an individual trait. According to the buffer hypothesis, certain factors can protect an older person when facing adversity or loss. For instance, having a supportive partner, a positive attitude toward close relationships, and social support may sustain well-being in the face of adversity.

In studying resilience, three essential elements need to be established: the exposure to stressors or adversities, a positive adaptive response or avoidance of negative outcomes, and the resources or mechanisms facilitating positive adaptation [21]. What constitutes an adversity or a stressor and how to determine positive adaptation can vary. When protecting factors or positive outcomes, it is necessary to consider the population studied and the severity of the adversity. Resilience research aims to produce information about utilizing resources as the adaptive mechanisms leading to positive outcomes. The manifestation of resilience varies across the life course, and less is known about resilience in older age compared to childhood and adolescence [21]. Challenges distinct to old age include lower physical functional capacity. On the other hand, earlier life experiences may provide resources that facilitate overcoming adversities. In different ages, similar adversity may be perceived differently.

Resilience research related to older individuals has mainly addressed long-term and cumulative adversities such as caregiving, cognitive and physical decline, or financial problems. There are also some recent studies examining transient or short-term adversities. For instance, in our study, physical functioning was examined as a factor protecting against health decline following a bone fracture [11]. Fractures are severe injuries causing substantial stress on an older human body and requiring considerable resources for recovery. We found that higher muscle strength and faster walking speed assessed before a fracture occurred were crucial in protecting against mortality after the fracture. The survival advantage among those with higher physical functioning was observed to be more extensive during the first year after a fracture than at other times. This indicated that good muscle strength and walking speed serve as indicators of reserves that can be utilized in times of crisis. We then studied also whether living with somebody vs. living alone would yield similar benefits when recuperating from a fracture. However, no difference in survival between those living alone vs. those living with somebody was observed during the years following the fracture [11, 12]. This was somewhat surprising as we expected that cohabiting would provide social resources buffering against health decline. When we looked into more detail at those living alone, we observed that in our data they represented higher socioeconomic position, were more active, and had more friends than those living with somebody, which we assumed may explain the result.

Recently an opportunity to study reduced possibilities for activities of choice as an adversity presented itself in the form of social distancing during the COVID-19 pandemic. Blocked possibilities to take part in meaningful activities potentially threaten quality of life, and the social distancing recommendations launched during the first wave of COVID-19 pandemic were considered the adversity [13]. We defined as the positive adaption the maintenance of high quality of life. The resources supporting positive adaptation were higher walking speed, absence of loneliness, living arrangement (living alone vs. with a partner), and stress-coping ability. Altogether 685community-dwelling 75–85-year-old persons were interviewed and examined in 2017–2018 and were followed by mailed questionnaires during COVID-19 social distancing in the spring of 2020. We set a cutoff for "constant high" quality of life based on staying in the highest baseline quartile over the follow-up. Perceived restrictiveness of the social distancing recommendations was recorded. Better stress-coping ability and not being lonely increased the odds for constant high quality of life from before to amid social distancing, and the odds did not differ according to the perceived restrictiveness of the social distancing recommendations. Higher walking speed predicted constant high quality of life only among those perceiving restrictiveness. Living arrangement was not associated with constant high quality of life. During social distancing, psychosocial resources helped to maintain good quality of life regardless of how restrictive the social distancing recommendations were perceived to be. Better physical capacity was important for constant high quality of life only among those perceiving restrictiveness presumably because it enabled replacing blocked indoor social activities with outdoor physical activities [13]. We concluded that maintaining a desired activity level by increasing outdoor exercise may have bestowed a sense of continuity while also manifesting further advantages, such as improved fitness and restorative experiences. Many older people do activities that take place at home (e.g., crafting, DIY, gardening). Such activities were not affected by the social distancing recommendations, and consequently people inclining to them did not need to draw on extra individual functional resources to maintain their quality of life.

Even though resilience in old age has limits, most older people can perceive good quality of life throughout late adulthood and old age even though objective circumstances might be unfavorable. Staudinger and Grevel [20] suggest that mastering adversities does not require special person-specific skills or conditions that are available to only a few certain individuals. They state that different constellations of resources, such as goal-oriented approach, skills, and compensatory strategies accumulated over lifetime, and searching of social support may make up resilience for different persons but even for one person across time or across different domains of functioning.

4.5 Adaptation in Old Age as the Foundation of Resilience

Gerontological research that has explored the adaptation processes in aging has laid the groundwork for the conceptualization of resilience. In addition to referring to adjusting to changes, adaptation refers to proactively shaping one's development using strategies encompassing goal engagement and goal disengagement and applying these strategies to shape one's environment according to their goals. Adaptation refers to a process of optimizing the fit between a person and the environment when faced with internal or external changes.

One of the first studies on stress and adaption in old age suggested that many potential stressors have less serious long-term outcomes than crisis orientation approach would suggest [18]. There are several theoretical approaches that concentrate on specific domains or levels of functioning, such as psychological or physiological adaptation. The resilience framework seeks to unite and underscore the significance of these diverse aspects for adaptation in old age.

Salutogenesis and Psychological Perspectives Resilience in later life is theoretically rooted in the model of salutogenesis by Professor Aaron Antonovsky in the late 1970s. It aims to explain why some people become unwell when exposed to stress and others do not. The central concept in the explanation is the sense of coherence, which describes whether life is understood as comprehensive, meaningful, and manageable [1]. Comprehensibility relates to the cognitive aspect and refers to the extent to which events can be rationally discerned in a structured way. The behavioral aspect—manageability—points to the degree of having resources to deal with the events. Meaningfulness describes the motivational aspect that we draw from when facing challenges and refers to the perceived emotional meaning of one's life.

A strong sense of coherence helps the individual to tap into resources that help identifying and using generalized and specific resistance resources. For example, in a study among family caregivers of persons with dementia, an intervention fostering sense of coherence improved mental well-being, and the positive influences were mediated through improved sense of coherence [23]. Family caregivers for a person with dementia often encounter psycho-behavioral symptoms related to dementia and exhibit increased risk of chronic stress, depressed mood, cognitive decline, and poor physical health than non-carers.

Antonovsky suggested that sense of coherence continues to develop until approximately age 30 and that it is maintained throughout adult life, but after retirement the sense of coherence diminishes. However, subsequent empirical research has not supported the idea that sense of coherence declines in older ages. Instead, sense of coherence may strengthen over the entire lifetime providing improved resources for coping with stressful life situations.

Aligned with salutogenesis, theories from positive and developmental psychology underpin resilience. Positive psychology emphasizes the constructive traits and strengths of individuals, such as optimism and engagement, in achieving well-being. Developmental psychology theories focus on adaptation through balancing gains and losses across different life phases.

Physiological Perspectives The physiological perspective of resilience examines the body's biological, physiological, and physical adaptation. Ferrucci et al. [6] propose a hierarchical model of aging metrics, highlighting the role of biological resilience mechanisms in maintaining dynamic equilibrium of intrinsic capacities. Functional aging begins when lower-level resilience mechanisms are depleted, impacting the body's ability to respond to stressors. Reserve capacity, created during lifespan developmental processes, is central to physical resilience. It described the potential of cells, tissues, or organs to function beyond their basal level in response to physiological demands.

We utilized a network approach for understanding intrinsic capacity as a system underlying functioning [14]. The system's resilience to resist functional decline may arise from the interrelationships among system components, i.e., body functions or capacities. We investigated whether the interplay between different capacities diverge according to age and self-rated health (SRH) in older adults. We quantified five capacity domains, vitality, locomotion, cognition, psychology, and sensory, using performance-based measurements and questionnaires. The capacity network density was higher in the older (80–85 years) vs. younger (75 years) individuals and in the worse compared to the better self-rated health group in both sexes. We concluded that with increasing age and health decline, the networks of bodily capacities become denser, which may indicate a loss of system resilience. In a dense system pathway, unfavorable changes in functional capacity can spread more rapidly from one system to another, and eventually the system may reach a tipping point and collapse. This phenomenon is most likely related to a decline in functional reserves [14].

Life Course Perspectives Aging and resilience manifestation in later life are part of a continuum influenced by earlier life phases, experiences, and exposures. Life course theories examine developmental pathways of resilience, considering interactions between individuals and environmental factors throughout life. Cumulative advantage and disadvantage theory suggests that exposures across the life course shape resilience, influencing how individuals adapt to stressors. The sensitive period model posits that exposures during critical life phases may have enduring consequences on later-life health and well-being. Life course studies are discussed in more detail in Chap. 9.

Socioecological Perspectives Socioecological models offer a comprehensive interdisciplinary perspective on adaptation processes during aging within the context of person-environment interactions. The ecological model of aging by Lawton and Nahemow [15] illustrates the balance between individual needs and environmental demands, emphasizing the achievement of optimal functioning through person-environment fit. Resilience models rooted in socioecological frameworks aim to capture the complex interactions between individuals and multilevel environmental factors, though empirical research in this area remains limited.

References

1. Antonovsky A. Health, stress and coping. San Francisco: Jossey-Bass; 1979.
2. Atchley RC. Continuity theory and the evolution of activity in later adulthood. In: Kelly JR, editor. Activity and aging: staying involved in later life. Sage; 1993. p. 5–16.
3. Baltes PB, Baltes MM. Psychological perspectives on successful aging: the model of selective optimization with compensation. In: Baltes PB, Baltes MM, editors. Successful aging: perspectives from the behavioral sciences. New York: Cambridge University Press; 1990. p. 1–34.
4. Cumming E, Henry WE. Growing old, the process of disengagement. Basic Books; 1961.
5. Deci EL, Ryan RM. Intrinsic motivation and self-determination in human behavior. New York: Plenum; 1985.
6. Ferrucci L, Levine ME, Kuo PL, Simonsick EM. Time and the metrics of aging. Circ Res. 2018;123:740–4.
7. Havighurst RJ. Successful aging. The Gerontologist. 1961;1:8–13.
8. Havighurst RJ, Albrecht R. Older people. New York: Longmans, Green; 1953.
9. Havighurst RJ, Neugarten BL, Tobin SS. Disengagement, personality and life satisfaction in the later years. University of Chicago; 1964.
10. Katz S. Critical gerontology for a new era. The Gerontologist. 2019;59:396–7.
11. Koivunen K, Sillanpää E, von Bonsdorff M, et al. Mortality risk among older people who did versus did not sustain a fracture: baseline prefracture strength and gait speed as predictors in a 15-year follow-up. J Gerontol A Biol Sci Med Sci. 2020a;75:1996–2002.
12. Koivunen K, Sillanpää E, von Bonsdorff M, et al. Living alone vs. living with someone as a predictor of mortality after a bone fracture in older age. Aging Clin Exp Res. 2020b;32:1697–705.
13. Koivunen K, Portegijs E, Sillanpää E, et al. Maintenance of high quality of life as an indicator of resilience during COVID-19 social distancing among community-dwelling older adults in Finland. Qual Life Res. 2022;31:713–22.
14. Koivunen K, Lindeman K, Välimaa M, et al. Investigating resilience through intrinsic capacity networks in older adults. J Gerontol A Biol Sci Med Sci. 2024;15:glae048.
15. Lawton MP, Nahemow L. Ecology and the aging process. In: Eisdorfer C, Lawton MP, editors. The psychology of adult development and aging. Washington, DC: American Psychological Association; 1973. p. 619–74.
16. Luthar SS, Cicchetti D, Becker B. The construct of resilience: a critical evaluation and guidelines for future work. Child Dev. 2000;71:543–62.

17. Masten AS. Ordinary magic: resilience processes in development. Am Psychol. 2001;2001(56):227–38.
18. Palmore E, Cleveland WP, Nowlin NB, et al. Stress and adaptation in later life. J Gerontol. 1979;34:841–51.
19. Rowe JW, Kahn RL. Successful aging. Gerontologist. 1997;37:433–40.
20. Staudinger UM, Grevel W. Resilience and aging. In: Pachana NA, editor. Encyclopedia of geropsychology. Singapore: Springer; 2017.
21. Windle G, Bennett KM, Noyes J. A methodological review of resilience measurement scales. Health Qual Life Outcomes. 2011;9:8.
22. World Health Organization. Active ageing: A policy framework. Geneva: Switzerland; 2002.
23. Yu DSF, Cheng ST, Chow EO, Kwok T, McCormack B, Wu W. The effects of a salutogenic strength-based intervention on sense of coherence and health outcomes of dementia family carers: a randomized controlled trial. Age. Aging. 2023;52:afad160.

Active Aging

5

Abstract

The framework of active aging gained importance in positive gerontology in the 2000s. The novelty was contesting the traditional view that associates the oldest stage of life with inactivity. World Health Organization published the policy framework for active aging. The United Nations Economic Commission for Europe (UNECE) initiated the Active Aging Index project. Subsequently, several suggestions were made about how to translate the active aging policy goals to pertain to individuals living their lives. Finally, this chapter presents a quantifiable active aging assessment tool pertaining to individuals.

5.1 Development and Operationalization of the Concept of Active Aging

There has been a surge in interest in the concept of active aging as a framework for understanding and promoting well-being among older adults. However, there appears to be conceptual confusion in the use of the word "activity" and with the concept of active aging. Sometimes the factors underlying active aging, the outcomes of active aging, and the active aging process itself are presented in commotion. The goal of this chapter is to present recent developments in active aging research and provide an outline for research.

In 2002, the World Health Organization published a health policy definition of active aging. According to this definition, countries and communities should "optimize older people's opportunities for health, participation, and security to ensure the highest quality of life for them." The World Health Organization further elaborated on this concept, defining active aging as a continuous pursuit of health, participation, and security to enhance the quality of life in older age [17]. This

T. Rantanen, *Advancing Research on Active Aging and Participation*,
https://doi.org/10.1007/978-3-031-94702-5_5

policy also emphasizes that societal measures should align with the preferences and goals of older people. Subsequently, active aging concept was further developed by the European Union as "empowering individuals to maintain control over their lives as they age, actively contributing to both the economy and society". The WHO definition of active aging exhibits the following chief properties (presented by São José and Teixeira [3] and São José et al. cited in [14]):

(a) Active aging is conceived as a collective responsibility, i.e., a societal responsibility, rather than an individual responsibility.
(b) Active aging should respect the older persons' preferences, needs, and capacities.
(c) Active aging should be achievable for all, also for older persons who are frail, disabled, and in need of care.
(d) Active aging comprises multiple activities (physical and mental, productive and non-productive).
(e) Active aging is a process that occurs throughout life (the life course perspective).
(f) The ultimate goal of active aging is to enhance older persons' quality of life.
(g) Active aging is shaped by several factors (economic, social, political).

The WHO policy goal emphasizes participation while the European union emphasizes autonomy and productivity in their definitions.

The WHO definition has gained some research interest, but the early attempts to operationalize it failed. For example, some researchers sought to categorize individuals and, in a sense, define an active aging phenotype based on the WHO definition. It appears that trying to model active aging as a trait or a phenotype that is present in some and not in others will lead to defective approaches. Some attempts have been made to validate an empirical model of an active aging phenotype based on the WHO definition by using, for example, latent factor analysis in survey data. However, the authors concluded that it was not possible to create a statistical model of WHO active aging definition that would fit their data (e.g., [2, 9]). Subsequently, a proposition of individual level active aging phenotype named following characteristics as features typical for active aging individuals: the maintenance of positive subjective well-being; good physical, social, and mental health; good functional ability and fitness; and continued involvement in one's family, peer group, and community throughout the aging process [4]. This definition has been criticized for being much too ambitious, normative, and possible only for very few. In my view, health, fitness, and functional abilities are relevant for active aging, but based on them, people's active aging level cannot be quantified. Rather they are predictors or consequences of active aging.

Central to the WHO framework is the notion of ongoing engagement adapted to individual needs and capacities. The WHO definition does not refer to active aging as a *state* of well-being. It is not a definition of an active aging phenotype but conveys the importance on promoting circumstances that allow older people to strive for well-being and good quality of life through their activities and participation in meaningful life situations. It rather implies that active aging is a process where engagements may change as preferences, goals, and resources of older people change. More importantly, the WHO definition cannot be directly applied to assess individuals. To assess the active aging of individuals, we first need to translate the policy definition to center on the individual to capture how the policies, when realized to a certain level, could interact with the lived experience of older adults.

There is still a great deal of ambiguity on what active aging is. Active aging as a concept has been criticized for being positioned as the ideal model for aging [16]. The concept of active aging highlights activity and the participation of older people in the society. However, this may lead to picture older adults as either active and independent or as frail, passive, dependent, and even a burden. There are disputes that active aging is somehow opposite to or dismissive of care needs and that it undermines the importance of care provision in the context of aging policy.

Having care needs does not exclude an active engagement in life that contributes to one's own well-being and the well-being of others. An example comes from our randomized controlled trial examining the effect of an outdoor activities' intervention delivered by older volunteers on the quality of life of those being served. The participants receiving help from the volunteers were older people with severe mobility limitations. The idea underlying the study was the observation that older people with severe mobility limitations have only limited possibilities for restorative activities. To compensate for this deficiency, we wanted to introduce new resources in the form of an outdoor activities buddy. This was a well-founded solution, because many participants could not access the outdoors without help of another person. In our intervention, the volunteer helped the participants access outdoors once a week to destinations according to the participants' wishes, which could be visiting the cemetery, buying a lottery ticket at a kiosk, seeing an art exhibition, or sitting on a bench in a nearby park. We observed that the relationships of the volunteer-participant dyads became reciprocal, and the participants receiving help contributed significantly to the activity accomplishments. The reciprocal social interaction co-created positive experiences and well-being for both the volunteering helper and the person being helped.

Active aging has been associated with the third age, which entails agency, sustained consumption, and living without assistance or daily care. Another related concept is productive aging, which is more focused on productive or useful activities, such as civil society participation, volunteer work, or work for pay. From that perspective, active aging is closely related to policies concerning labor force participation of older people. Older adults will be encouraged to work longer, volunteer, follow a healthy lifestyle, and prepare for aging [17]. In state policies, active aging has indeed been dominated by a rather narrow financial interpretation that highlights the extension of working life to reduce "the burden" of population aging and provide a reservoir of labor force (discussed in more detail in Chap. 10). Another context where the term active aging is frequently used, however usually not defined, concerns health technology, pharmaceuticals, and care provision enterprises, all of which have high financial interests. Their interpretations of active aging may be overselling the potential of their products for disability prevention and management, and thus they represent a narrow view of active aging. In all, there is a need for a more comprehensive approach to active aging.

While promoting individuality and distinctiveness in its emphasis on goals and preferences, active aging research also needs to acknowledge that people function in a context and possess different resources. Active aging should be viewed inclusive in terms that it concerns frail, disabled, healthy, and vigorous people. Active aging policy actions should enable and promote preferred ways of engagement for people of all functional abilities. The concept of active aging entails the actions that people take to promote well-being for themselves and others based on their goals and opportunities. Empirical studies have demonstrated a positive correlation between increased activity levels and enhanced well-being in later life (e.g., [5, 8]). Despite the widespread use of active aging concept, there remains a lack of consensus on how to operationalize and measure active aging at the individual level in an inclusive way while also considering the diversity of older age groups.

5.2 What Is Activity?

Activity refers to everything that people do. Human activity encompasses a broad spectrum of actions beyond mere physical movements. The word activity covers meaningful engagement in social, economic, and cultural activities, family life, volunteering, paid work, and physical activity. These activities may include tasks related to health and self-care, social interactions, the upkeep of one's living environment, or political activism. Being active is central to human behavior. People are by nature inclined to participate in activities that they find appealing, enjoyable, and fulfilling or their duty. Intrinsic motivation propels engagement in activities that yield enjoyment and satisfaction. This type of motivation is characterized by a genuine interest in the activity itself, without any external contingencies influencing the person's engagement [12]. However, people also do various activities for being socially desirable or repaid, in which case external pressures, necessities, or rewards drive the motivation.

The WHO hosted an extensive consultation process among top scientists to come up with a meaningful system to categorize activities and participation similarly to disease categorization. The result was the International Classification of Functioning, Disability and Health (ICF) in 2001. This is discussed in more detail in Sect. 6.4.

I suggest that in the context of active aging, activities should be described based on their *purpose* rather than external criteria. The purpose of an activity may stay unchanged while the way or intensity of the activity is adapted to personal situation. The activities requiring physical force will change with increasing age even though their purpose remain the same. Long hikes on the mountains may transform into strolls in the park. Nevertheless, meeting the purpose of the activity may restore a sense of well-being even though its concrete forms may have changed. Some confusion in active aging research stems from conceptual incoherence that fails to differentiate circumstances or affordances for and consequences of activity from activity itself. In the discussion about active aging sometimes the elements of active aging are confused with its correlates or underlying factors.

5.3 The Active Aging Index

The Active Aging Index project was initiated by the United Nations Economic Commission for Europe (UNECE), the European Commission's Director General for Employment, Social Affairs and Inclusion, and the European Centre for Social Welfare Policy and Research in Vienna [1, 18]. The index is used in the European Union, but also in other countries outside of it. The index being an "evidence-based tool" can be used to monitor, compare, promote, and indicate the activity of older adults in different countries and to produce knowledge to develop policymaking [1].

The Active Aging Index consists of four domains: employment; participation in society; independent, healthy, and secure living; and capacity and enabling environment for active aging. The "employment" domain contains information about employment rate at different ages up to 74 years. The "participation in society" domain includes data on volunteering, care of children and grandchildren, care of disabled, and political participation. The domain of "independent, healthy and secure living" includes items such as physical exercise, access to health services, independent living, financial security, physical safety, and lifelong learning. The domain "capacity and enabling environment" incorporates data on remaining life expectancy and share of healthy life expectancy at different ages, mental well-being, use of ICT, social connectedness, and educational attainment.

The criticisms of the AAI include its lack of theoretical depth and for being focused predominantly on productive activities. In addition, the index does not acknowledge what activities are personally important to older adults. AAI is meant for evaluating countries. Some of its items are meaningless in the context of individuals, such as life expectancy or employment rate, which are population-based estimates.

Recently, a qualitative study used AAI as the framework for their analyses on active aging of older adults who need care and services, the fourth agers. Kiuru and Valokivi [6] wanted to assess the relevance of the AAI domains in the lives of older frail people. The domains of "independent, healthy and secure living" and "capacity and enabling environment for active aging" were most common in their data, while the domain of "*participation in society*" was quite rare. The participants needed help themselves, and political activity was more about following politics. The domain of "independent, healthy and secure living" was present widely in the participants' lives. The authors noticed that participants did things independently, but also received help to stay active. Participants placed high value on taking care of physical health and the ability to move. The participants used health and social care services, but independent living was important for them. The participants did things like going to places, doing housework, running errands, and taking care of personal hygiene as independently as possible. Matters concerning *financial security* overlapped with independent living when participants talked about their use of money and help with managing it. The "use of ICT" was not common among the participants. When it came to educational attainment, the participants had studied in the old model of primary school, or had vocational training, and had worked in jobs that were rather physically demanding, such as cleaning, farming, or logging. Life expectancy and healthy life expectancy was frequently in the participants' thoughts in terms of own or family members' future. A remarkable result of this study concerns activities that were *not* covered in AAI but that were considered important for well-being. The participants reported diverse hobbies and interests, such as karaoke, handcrafts, watching TV, feeding birds, and reading. Other things that the participants mentioned were various chores, naps, eating, and just hanging out. The passage of time was important for the participants. Continuing personal routines, working on small tasks, and just living a "regular life" were important for their well-being [6].

Many older people wish to remain active through engagement in a variety of activities, even small activities, regardless of being in less-than-perfect health. While the AAI may be suitable for assessing the active aging situation at the state or community level, it cannot be applied in individual-level research, and it fails to capture the essential daily activities that propel a sense of being a player in one's own life.

5.4 Active Aging as Lived Experience

One of the first scales developed to assess active aging of individual people and to conceptually structure the concept of active aging originates from Thailand. This scale was developed in a multi-phase process including qualitative interviews among older people, expert panel discussions, focus groups, feedback interviews among older people, statistical analyses of quantitative data, and psychometric analyses of the scale properties. The result was the Active Aging Scale-Thai (AAS-Thai) which assesses the multidimensional nature of active aging or the process of being actively engaged in life as one grows old. It includes seven subscales and altogether 36 items. The subscales were named with respect to the process of being actively engaged in life: (1) being self-reliant, (2) being actively engaged with society, (3) developing spiritual wisdom, (4) building up financial security, (5) maintaining a healthy lifestyle, (6) engaging in active learning, and (7) strengthening family ties with respect to being cared for in late life [15].

Being self-reliant includes eight items representing a person's ability to independently take care of their self and includes tasks related to family-care. Being actively engaged with society incorporates eight items, including engaging in social participation and social contribution. Developing spiritual wisdom involves having inner strength and calmness, including trusting in religion, and making merits. Building up financial security was characterized as preparing financially for later life and for funerary activities as well as having enough money for daily expenses. Maintaining a healthy lifestyle incorporates health-promoting behaviors, such as eating healthy food and practicing physical activity or exercise. Engaging in active learning reflects the capacity to learn about new information technologies to make one cognitively active and healthy. Strengthening family ties to ensure care in later life includes items like strengthening family ties and teaching children about filial piety. This dimension concerns activities of parents to ensure that their children will care for them when they are old or frail [15].

The progressive features of AAS-Thai include that the items indicate activity that has specific purpose without quantifying the level of doing the activity. It does not solely concentrate on circumstances or consequences of active aging. It is a quantifiable measure that can be used as an outcome or as a predictor in studies on well-being of older people. The subscales describe active endeavor and strive to using own actions reach specific goals that represent active aging for the participants, i.e., activities that they undertake to promote well-being.

5.5 Developing The University of Jyväskylä Active Aging Scale (UJACAS)

To enable research on active aging pertaining to individuals, we started to develop the concept of active aging at individual level as lived life while emphasizing older adults' active involvement in their daily lives. We aimed at assessing active aging as the extent to which individuals pursue activities that resonate with their personal goals, functional abilities, and available opportunities [11]. Unlike the traditional model of successful aging put forth by Rowe and Kahn [13], which primarily focuses on health as the outcome, active aging emphasizes a dynamic process that accommodates individuals with limitations and disabilities while considering their own preferences [10]. Therefore, the question arises: What does the life of an older individual look like if the policy goal of active aging is achieved? While some definitions of active aging closely resemble those of successful aging, focusing on aspects like physical fitness and cognitive function, they often overlook the importance of meaningful engagement in later life [4]. Additionally, equating active aging solely with physical activity fails to capture the diverse range of activities older adults may find fulfilling.

In response to these challenges, we proposed a new definition of active aging emphasizing the pursuit of promoting good quality of life through activities aligned with personal goals, functional capacities, and opportunities [11]. This inclusive approach acknowledges the diversity of experiences among older adults, including also those with disabilities and limitations (Table 5.1). The novelty of this definition is that it centers on an individual and assesses the lived experience of older people. Drawing on the COM-B system [7], which posits that health behavior (B) is influenced by capability (C), opportunity (O), and motivation (M), our definition

Table 5.1 The World Health Organization definition of active aging and how it can be translated to concern the lived experience of older people

World Health Organization policy definition of active aging	Translation into lived experience of older people
"… the process of optimizing opportunities for health, participation, and security in order to enhance quality of life as people age. These policies should be in line with the needs, preferences and capacities of older people…"	"Striving of older people for Well-being through activity according to their goals, capabilities, and available opportunities."

incorporates four key aspects: willingness, ability, autonomy, and activity. We defined active aging as the *striving of older people for well-being through activity according to their goals, abilities, and available opportunities.*

To permit empirical research, we created a quantitative questionnaire assessing active aging [11] that comprised four aspects of each activity: goals, abilities, opportunities, and activity. Goals refer to how much one wanted to do the activity. Ability refers to being able to do the activity. When assessing their opportunities, people evaluate their affordances to the specific activity, i.e., what their environment offers in terms of undertaking the task they wish to perform and whether they have ties or responsibilities that prevent them from doing the activity or facilitate doing the activity. Finally, activeness was quantified by the participants evaluating the degree or frequency of doing each activity. The underlying idea is that people of all ages naturally strive to promote their well-being through their own activity in their current situation in life, as proposed in the self-determination theory.

To create a quantifiable scale, we first needed to develop a list of activities in essential life areas. We took as our starting point the "Activities and Participation" categories of the International Classification of Functioning, Disability and Health ("Towards a Common Language for Functioning, Disability and Health, ICF," 2002, accessed 20.10.2024) which provides a valid, well-thought-out classification of essential life areas. In this classification, activity is defined as an execution of a task or action by an individual. Participation refers to involvement in a life situation. There are nine subcategories in the "Activities and Participation" category. The subcategories are as follows: 1. learning and applying knowledge, 2. general tasks and demands, 3. communication, 4. mobility, 5. self-care, 6. domestic life, 7. interpersonal interactions and relationships, 8. major life areas, and 9. community, social, and civic life. The ICF categorizations refer to abilities or limitations in doing the tasks, but we wanted to express them as doings and phrased them in the manner that indicates pursuing something. In our scale, a good example of active agency in doing something concerns interpersonal relations. Probably the most widely used approach to studying interpersonal relations of older people is to enquire whether they suffer from loneliness. In UJACAS the items of interpersonal relationships concern helping others, taking actions to maintain friendships, and taking actions to learn to know new people, i.e., positive actions that people take to promote their social relationships.

For each item, we formulated questions from four aspects:

1. Willingness to do the activity (how much have you in the past 4 weeks wanted to…).
2. Opportunity to do the task (during past 4 weeks have you had the opportunity to…).
3. Ability to do the task (during the past 4 weeks, have you been able to…).
4. Frequency of the activity (during the past for weeks how often have you done...)

In the scale creation process, a group of researchers came up with ideas about activities to be included in the scale. Initially, the list was long and was iterated several times making use of comments of older pilot respondents. Subsequently, the scale was refined and validated in a multiphase process. The draft scale was tested in a pilot study for item analysis and scale validity. A feedback study with focus groups and questionnaire respondents provided input about the phrasing and meaningfulness of the items. The reliability was then assessed in a test-retest study.

The result was a 17-item University of Jyvaskyla Active Aging Scale with four aspects in each item (goals, ability, opportunity, and activity; score range 0–272). The psychometric and item properties are good, and the scale was found to assess a unidimensional latent construct of active aging [11]. Eight of the ICF subcategories were covered in our scale, but no items in the sub-category communication were included in the final version of the scale. Please see Table 5.2 for included items.

During the scale creation process, we elaborated several items that were perceived as vague or biased and rejected several items that might appear intuitively important for active aging. For example, we first phrased an item on spirituality as

Table 5.2 The UJACAS items included in the final scale according to the ICF categories of activities and participation

ICF activities and participation category	UJACAS item
Learning and applying knowledge	Practicing memory; using computer
General tasks and demands	Advancing matters in own life
Mobility	Exercising; enjoying the outdoors
Self-care	Taking care of appearance
Domestic life	Crafting or DIY; making home cozy and pleasant
Interpersonal interactions	Helping others; maintaining friendships; getting to know new people
Major life areas	Balancing personal economics; making one’s days interesting
Community, social, and civic life	Practicing artistic hobbies like singing or painting; participating in events; advancing societal/communal matters; doing things according to one’s conviction or world view

"Acting according to spiritual or religious conviction." The feedback from the focus group suggested that religiosity was too prominent in this item. Subsequently, the final formulation was "Taking actions to promote matters in accordance with my faith or worldview." An example of rejected items concerns teaching and advising others, which we felt might indicate generativity. However, the older participants considered this socially problematic and vague, and the item was rephrased to helping and supporting others. Items were rejected if they were considered vague or irrelevant by our participants or if they did not contribute to the variability of the scale based on item analyses. We also went through several options for formulating the questions in the subscale of goals. First, we asked the participants how important they considered an activity to be for them. This resulted in practically no variability in responses, as all the activities were considered generally important even though the participants did not necessarily consider them priorities for themselves. Eventually, we formulated the subscale "how much you have wanted to do (this activity)" as it better reflects personal motivation to be active in the specific pursuits (see [11] for description of the process).

The scale is designed for use among older individuals who can provide independent responses. It is not restricted to any specific subset of the older population. We have successfully conducted interviews among diverse participants, spanning from residents of assisted living facilities to highly active individuals living independently within their communities. To ensure comprehensive reporting, we have set the recall period for 4 weeks, allowing adequate time to account for any exceptional circumstances that may have occurred during the preceding weeks, such as unusual weather conditions, illness, travel, or infrequent social engagements. This scale effectively distinguishes between respondents who are more active from those who are less active. Validation analyses indicate that higher scores on the scale correlate with more favorable outcomes, though the nature of the association—whether linear or, for instance, curved—in relation to indicators of well-being, warrants further investigation. The UJACAS scale and its assessment notes are presented in Attachment 1. at the end of this book. Predictors and consequences of active aging will be discussed more detail in Chap. 7.

References

1. AAI in brief. AAI project, joint project by the United Nations economic Commission for Europe (UNECE) and the European Commission. https://statswiki.unece.org/display/AAI/I.+AAI+in+brief (2021). Accessed 20 Jan 2025.
2. Bélanger E, Ahmed T, Filiatrault J, et al. An empirical comparison of different models of active aging in Canada: the international mobility in aging study. The Gerontologist. 2017;57:197–205.
3. de São José J, Teixeira AR. Envelhecimento ativo: contributo para uma discussão crítica. Análise Social. 210;2014;28–54 XLIX (1.º).
4. Fernández-Ballesteros R, Robine JM, Walker A, et al. Active aging: a global goal. Curr Gerontol Geriatr Res. 2013;2013:298012.
5. Guell C, Shefer G, Griffin S, et al. 'Keeping your body and mind active': an ethnographic study of aspirations for healthy ageing. BMJ Open. 2016;6:e009973.

6. Kiuru H, Valokivi H. "I do those things to pass the time": active aging during fourth age. J Aging Stud. 2022;61:101037.
7. Michie S, van Stralen MM, West R. The behaviour change wheel: a new method for characterising and designing behaviour change interventions Implement Sci 2011;6;1; https://doi.org/10.1186/1748-5908-6-42.
8. Paggi ME, Jopp D, Hertzog C. The importance of leisure activities in the relationship between physical health and wellbeing in a life span sample. Gerontology. 2016;62:450–8.
9. Paúl C, Ribeiro O, Teixeira L. Active ageing: an empirical approach to the WHO model. Curr Gerontol Geriatr Res. 2012;2012:382972.
10. Rantanen T, Äyräväinen I, Eronen J, et al. The effect of an outdoor activities' intervention delivered by older volunteers on the quality of life of older people with severe mobility limitations: a randomized controlled trial. Aging Clin Exp Res. 2015;27:161–9.
11. Rantanen T, Portegijs E, Kokko K, Rantakokko M, Törmäkangas T, Saajanaho M. Developing an assessment method of active aging: university of Jyvaskyla active aging scale. J Aging Health. 2019;31:1002–24.
12. Ryan RM, Deci EL. Self-determination theory and the facilitation of intrinsic motivation social development and well-being. Am Psychol. 2000;55;1:68–78. https://doi.org/10.1037/0003-066X.55.1.68.
13. Rowe J, Kahn R. Successful aging. New York: Random House; 1997.
14. São José JM, Timonen V, Amado CAF, et al. A critique of the active ageing index. J Aging Stud. 2017;40:49–56.
15. Thanakwang K, Isaramalai SA, Hatthakit U. Development and psychometric testing of the active aging scale for Thai adults. Clin Interv Aging. 2014;9:1211–21.
16. Timonen V. Beyond successful and active ageing: a theory of model ageing. Bristol: Policy Press; 2016.
17. World Health Organization. Towards a common language for functioning, disability and health. Geneva: ICF; 2002.
18. Zaidi A, Stanton D. Active aging index: analytical report. Brussels: UNECE and European Commission Directorate General for Employment, Social Affairs and Inclusion; 2015.

Functional Capacity, Activities, and Participation

6

Abstract

Functional capacity is a central indicator of health in old age because it reflects the severity of the chronic conditions and at the same time serves as a resource for participation in different life situations. Functioning of older people can be addressed from the point of view what they are physically or cognitively able to do and conversely what they are unable to do which refers to disability. There is no uniform way to categorize or outline functional capacity. Commonly used headings include activities of daily living (ADL), instrumental activities of daily living (IADL), and mobility. Autonomy in mobility is essential for the opportunity to lead a life the way one wants and participate in social activities and access community amenities. Models outlining different levels of functioning, such as cellular, organ, whole person, and person-environment interaction, help understand how more distal and proximal variables relate to disability outcomes. People cope with functional deficits in different ways that may be adaptive or maladaptive in the circumstances that they live considering that physical and social environment may support or hinder mobility.

When growing old, functional capacity and its changes reflect the consequences of diseases, treatments, aging process, and genetic dispositions. Functional capacity is a good indicator of health both at the individual and population levels. High functional capacity indicates a reserve that increases the likelihood of sustained functional independence even when facing stressors.

Functional capacity refers to how well and safely a person can perform tasks that are personally important, necessary, or their responsibilities. *Disability* means that the functional capacity, such as psychological or physical condition, is insufficient for social roles, striving for personal goals, or environmental demands. Disability is

T. Rantanen, *Advancing Research on Active Aging and Participation*, https://doi.org/10.1007/978-3-031-94702-5_6

typically manifested as difficulties or inability to do the task. Functional capacity develops and improves in youth, remains at a good relatively stable level through decades followed by a slight decline starting around 60–70 years of age. Subsequent more significant turn for the worse takes place about 10 years before death, with a steeper decline starting approximately 2 years before death.

Functional capacity can be categorized in various ways, but often the key areas include **personal roles, social roles, mobility, physical and cognitive capacity, and sensory functioning**. Functional capacity can be assessed through interviews and observations or by conducting tests and measurements.

Direct tests such as measured walking speed or hand grip strength provide standardized results that are useful for monitoring changes in the same individual, comparing differences between groups, or evaluating recovery among individuals receiving different treatments. The disadvantage of such measures is that they may not directly translate into how easily a person may carry out daily tasks. Instead, self-reports of functional capacity reflect a person's experience of how their functional capacity relates to the demands of their daily life or living environment. The downside is that difficulties in tasks such as bathing or walking may be related to features of the persons' residence or living environment, in addition to their physical functional capacity, making comparisons between different groups or countries problematic (Table 6.1).

Participation problems describe the consequences for individuals of the disparity between declining functional capacity and environmental demands and support. Participation refers to being involved in important life situations.

Table 6.1 Advantages and disadvantages of direct measures and self-reports in assessing functional capacity

Measurement type	Description	Advantages	Disadvantages
Direct measures	Standardized measurements like walking speed or hand grip strength can be used to monitor changes within individuals or differences between groups	Useful for tracking individual changes, comparing groups, or assessing recovery with different treatments	Results may not clearly indicate how they relate to everyday functioning or real-life activities
Self-reports of functional capacity	Reflect a person's experience of how their functional capacity interacts with the demands of their daily life or living environment	Provides insight into a person's subjective experience in relation to their environment	Environmental factors (e.g., home setup) can affect results, making cross-group or cross-country comparisons difficult and less reliable

6.1 Basic and Instrumental Activities of Daily Living

The most widely studied activities are related to personal roles and concern daily basic self-care activities, such as eating or bathing. These activities have been termed activities of daily living and abbreviated as *ADL*s. Assessing ADL functioning is part of care needs assessments. Difficulties in ADLs indicate such severe problems in functional capacity that independently getting through daily life is unlikely, and support and assistance are necessary. Activities related to managing various matters are referred to as instrumental activities of daily living (IADLs). Examples of instrumental activities include using the phone, cooking, or managing money. Almost all individuals with ADL impairments also have IADL impairments.

Daily basic functions are often assessed with questions based on the Katz ADL Index, which was developed by Dr. Sidney Katz in the early 1960s for various patient groups. The index evaluates the independent ability to perform tasks such as bathing, dressing, using the toilet, transferring from a chair or bed, maintaining continence, and eating. The response options in the original scale were "independently" and "not independently." Initially, the index was primarily used to assess patients' needs for assistance when being discharged from hospital care. In 1965, physiotherapist Dorothea Barthel published her own functional assessment tool, the Barthel Index, which was specifically used to evaluate the independent functional capacity of stroke patients. The Barthel Index includes ten functions, with additional items related to mobility that were not in Katz's index. The assessment can be conducted through self-report or observation. Each section is classified into three categories: unable, independent, and needs assistance. Similar types of categories are still used today, and their application has expanded to population studies. For example, according to the Finnish Institute for Health and Welfare's Finsote study, 11% of Finns over the age of 75 experience significant difficulties with ADL activities. However, the age category of over 75 is not very informative in itself, as it spans an age range of about 30 years, and ADL difficulties likely accumulate in the upper part of the age distribution.

Mapping basic daily tasks now forms a part of nearly all health and functional assessment tools. The Resident Assessment Instrument (RAI) is in use in many countries as an instrument to help develop the quality of long-term care of older people. Nowadays, the assessment of an individual's care needs has expanded to cover aspects related to the environment and participation. The evaluation questions cover the following areas: health status, functional ability, medication, nutrition, cognitive functions and mood, rehabilitation and special care, service usage, environment, participation and activity, and support from others.

Over the years, several tools have been developed to assess instrumental activities. The most widely used tool is the IADL scale (The Lawton Instrumental Activities of Daily Living Scale), developed by psychologist Mortimer Powell Lawton in collaboration with sociologist and social work researcher Elaine M. Brody. The scale was published in 1969 and was designed to evaluate the essential instrumental activities of older adults, such as managing finances, preparing meals, shopping, using the telephone, and managing medications or handling

Table 6.2 Summary of the central tenets of ADL and IADL assessments

Aspect	Details
Assessment methods of ADLs and IADLs	Self-reporting of difficulties, using proxy respondents (family/nurses), observing performance. Self-reports describe the respondents' immediate experience in the current circumstances
Observation	Observation can be used to assess independence and safety during task performance. Impairments, like balance issues, can raise concerns about safety while performing tasks
First noticeable signs of decline	Depend on the underlying diseases or injuries. Cognitive decline may manifest as difficulties in IADLs, such as difficulties in using a cellphone or online banking. Impairments in physical function, due to heart or musculoskeletal diseases, may manifest as avoidance of physically demanding tasks like long walks
Importance of ADLs and IADLs	Both are critical for maintaining independent living and evaluating needs for assistance

money. The purpose of the scale was to guide the identification of the most suitable living environment for an older person. The IADL assessment must consider prevailing gender roles and the era, as they are culturally bound. For example, using the telephone or managing finances is different today due to digitalization than what it was when the scale was developed. The scale is widely used, and in later versions the questions have been modified to measure the ability to perform the tasks, when necessary, rather than reflecting gender-specific habits (Table 6.2).

6.2 Social Roles and Activities

Social activity is an important aspect of life and a source of enjoyment. Being active in maintaining friendships, helping others, participating in organizations, attending cultural and sporting events, religious services, organizational events, going on trips, participating in social groups, and visiting relatives and friends are examples of social activity. Social activities help maintain a higher quality of life even when functional capacities decline.

The COVID-19 pandemic raised concerns about the older people's ability to maintain social contacts through internet applications, such as Skype, and several studies were conducted on that topic. We found in our study among 750 men and women aged 75 years and over that older adults show considerable diversity in their use of digital devices (computers, tablets, smart phones). Becoming a digital device user is a process, prompted by interest and motivation, leading to learning, either alone or with support from other people, and culminating in the adoption, in various ways, of information technology in one's everyday life [8].

Social activity refers to human interactions that take place in both informal and formal settings. Informal interactions include contacts via phone, letters, email, or social media, as well as in-person gatherings with family members, relatives, friends, and neighbors. Formal interactions, on the other hand, involve activities

Table 6.3 An example of categorizations of social activity and its benefits

Type of social participation	Description	Examples	Consequences/benefits
Collective social activity	Involves engaging with others in a community setting, focusing on personal development, socializing, and emotional support	Attending cultural events, traveling, group exercises, dancing, participating in organizations	Provides emotional support, sense of being liked, accepted, and understood. Correlated with a reduced risk of mortality and institutionalization in a 17-year follow-up study
Productive social activity	Focuses on contributing to others' Well-being or the common good, either through formal (volunteer work) or informal (helping others) contributions	Volunteer work, helping others informally	Promotes feelings of doing good, being useful, contributing to the common good, and reassurance of self-worth

such as attending organizational or club meetings, participating in religious services, and engaging in volunteer work. Another way to conceptually categorize social participation can be based on the content, context, and consequences of the activity. Collective social activity involves spending time and engaging with others, often as part of personal involvement in the community, where the individual's focus is on socializing and the interaction serves as a source of emotional support. Examples of collective social activities include attending cultural events, traveling, group exercises, dancing, and participating in organizational or congregational activities (Table 6.3). Productive social activity occurs when a person contributes to the well-being of others or the common good either formally, e.g., in a volunteer organization, or informally helping others. Collective social activities often provide a sense of being liked, accepted, and understood. Productive social activities can foster feelings of doing good, being useful, and contributing to a common good and provide experiences of reassurance of worth. In our follow-up study of approximately 17 years, we found that collective social activity correlated with a reduced risk of mortality and institutionalization, even when sociodemographic factors, health, functioning, and intensity of physical activity were controlled for [21].

6.3 Mobility

Moving outside the home supports participation in social life and enables access to many services and community amenities. The most common reasons for going outdoors among older people include shopping, walking for exercise, social visits, and running errands, i.e., activities that are essential or recreational.

A person's mobility is optimal when they can safely and reliably travel to where they want and when they want, and they can choose the mode of travel as they want [31]. Moving outdoors especially further away from home is often one of the first activities that older adults experience burdensome. The difficulties emerge when functional capacity gradually declines. Independent living may become cumbersome when a person cannot safely walk a distance of a few hundred meters, because the inability to walk safely increases the need of assistance also when trying to get into other modes of transportation, such as driving or using public transportation. According to the Finnish Institute of Health and Welfare, outdoor mobility difficulties are quite common among the people aged 75 years and over with 22% of men and 30% of women reporting difficulty walking 500 m (Results—THL, accessed 21.2. 2025); advanced mobility limitations are rather rare with the projected prevalence being about 7% [15].

The ability to move can be assessed, for example, by asking whether a person experiences difficulties in walking specific distances. Degree of difficulty in walking across a room, 100 m, 500 m, or 2 km, or climbing a flight of stairs are often recorded in epidemiological studies. Such knowledge provides a valid idea of the general functional capacity of a person while at the same time being technically easy to process. Another way to assess the ability to move is by conducting mobility tests. Commonly used tests include measuring walking speed, standing up from a chair, the 6-min walk test, or tests measuring balance. Measuring walking speed is easy to perform and requires only a stopwatch or light sensors and a marked distance on the floor. To ensure comparability, the measurement method should be standardized.

Key aspects of mobility include the mode of transport (e.g., driving, running, walking), the ability to move (e.g., being able to drive, run, walk), the extent of mobility (e.g., distance traveled, energy consumption for physical activity), patterns of activity (e.g., intensity, duration, fragmentation), and autonomy (e.g., satisfaction with mobility opportunities). Mobility can be studied from several perspectives (Table 6.4).

Sensory functions, balance, muscle strength, and the coordinating central nervous system are important for mobility. When moving the body in a specific direction, these systems collaborate. The ability to maintain physical activity for several minutes also depends on the respiratory and circulatory systems' ability to ensure

Table 6.4 Definitions of concepts related to mobility

Concept	What it means
Mobility	Includes all movement and traveling either by muscle power or also using vehicles
Life-space	Area where a person regularly moves
Autonomy in mobility	Satisfaction with opportunities to go to destinations outside the home
Physical activity	Voluntary muscle activity that increases energy expenditure and usually leads to movement
Exercise	Physical activity carried out for specific reasons or effects and usually as a hobby
Mobility capacity	Measured, observed, or perceived ability to move oneself or change body position

oxygen and energy supply. Because walking speed reflects the functioning of muscles, the balance system, the central nervous system, as well as the respiratory and circulatory systems, it is a valid predictor of health changes. In a large meta-analysis (nearly 15,000 participants), it was found that the risk of death for the lowest quartile of walking speed distribution was almost three times higher compared to the highest quartile [5].

In addition to self-report measures, the breadth of mobility has been studied recently using methods such as GPS tracking and accelerometers. Mobility can also be investigated by showing a map of places visited and reporting how one traveled there. Mobility activity within the life-space can also be explored through interviews.

Among older adults, walking, driving, and using public transport are the most common forms of independent and assisted mobility among older adults. Walking safely is essential for the use of other modes of transportation without assistance. Thus, the different modes of mobility may share similar determinants. To prevent people from becoming homebound, a situation that may eventually lead to marginalization from social activities, loneliness, and poor quality of life, better knowledge about the factors that hinder or support the independent community mobility of older people can promote active aging and reduce health disparities [26]. In the long term, most chronic conditions will encumber mobility through various mechanisms. The impairments most studied are those directly influencing walking: muscle strength and balance. However, impairments in vision and hearing may hinder the ability to divide attention while walking between traffic or having a conversation, for example, potentially increasing a risk for falls and other accidents. Co-existing vision, hearing, and balance impairments increased the risk of falls to almost 30-fold compared to people with no impairments [16].

The volume of mobility is a broader construct than physical activity because it also includes traveling by transportation. This can be illustrated with the concept of life-space. Life-space refers to the area in which a person moves as part of their everyday life. It includes the home, yard, neighborhood, city, or more distant areas. In old age, the life-space decreases, so that at its smallest, an older person's life-space may consist of only one room. Life-space and physical activity are related but not the same thing. Driving a car, for example, may compensate for deficits of the lower extremity performance and help maintain a wider life-space. Traveling by vehicle to the city center also increases physical activity because there may be walking involved at the destination. Our study Life-Space Mobility among Older People found that on days when older people did not leave their homes, they spent most of their time sitting and resting, and the level of physical activity was negligible. Leaving the house significantly increased physical activity [20].

Life-space mobility refers to the size of the spatial area (bedroom, home, outside home, neighborhood, town, distant locations; see Fig. 6.1) a person purposely moves through in daily life and to the frequency of travel within a specific time and need of assistance for that travel [1]. The first reports on life-space concerned nursing home residents, and later also community-living older people were targeted for life-space studies. Life-space can be used to assess transitions in independent living. Shrinking life-space signals giving up valued activities, such as social visits,

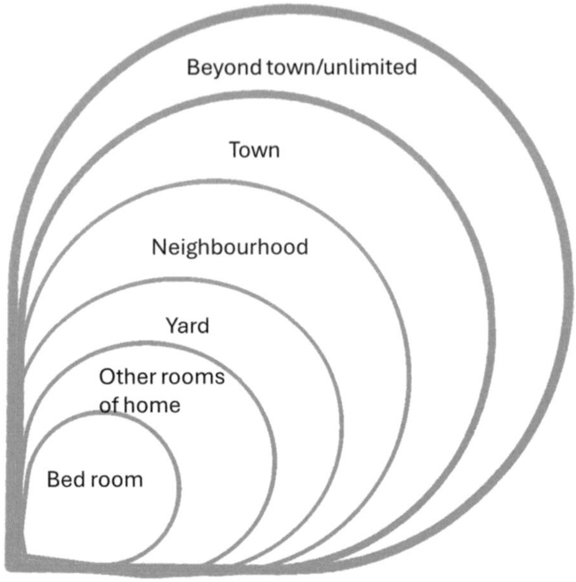

Fig. 6.1 A schematic figure of different levels of life-space. At its smallest, the life-space may comprise only of the bedroom. A slightly large life-space comprises also other rooms of the home. Outside home the yard, neighborhood and town form the following larger levels of life-space. Life-space mobility assessment factors in the levels visited, the frequency of these visits, and the assistance needed for going to different levels [1]

hobbies, recreation or work, and reduced use of community amenities, potentially lowering quality of life. We found that a large life-space is associated with good quality of life, but it does not guarantee it. A severely restricted life-space is consistently associated with low quality of life. Whether an older person regularly accesses vs. does not access the outdoors implies a lot about their life situation, physical activity, and their ability to participate in community life [23]. The risk factors underlying lower life-space mobility include higher age, lower socioeconomic status, and related health disparities such as higher body mass index, poorer cognitive capacity, and poorer physical performance [7].

Life-space mobility correlates with physical activity, but does not overlap with it completely. Going out of the home will increase physical activity. Activities done in multiple life-space areas contribute more to daily step counts than those done in fewer life-space levels. Shopping and walking for exercise, which are common reasons to go outdoors among community-dwelling older people contribute significantly to accumulation of physical activity assessed using wearable monitors [34].

6.4 Models of Disability Development and Participation

Aging and diseases accelerate the decline in functional capacity. In some cases, the decline is gradual and slow, while in others, a catastrophic event leads to a sudden decline in functional capacity. For example, the effects of a stroke or a bone fracture on functional capacity are immediate. In some other cases, the decline in functional capacity can take years, and it may be influenced by multiple diseases, unfavorable lifestyles, as well as problems related to the environment, poverty, or social relationships. In these situations, the factors and mechanisms underlying the decline in functional capacity may be difficult to crystallize.

A logical model of the relationships between different levels of variables may help to outline analyses of factors contributing to disablement. The benefit of models or outlines for different levels of functioning is that they organize the connections between dimensions of different levels of functional capacity and are thus helpful in structuring studies and analytical approaches in a cohesive manner.

The most used model in empirical research that categorizes factors contributing to the development of disabilities is based on the conceptual analysis Saad Nagi conducted in 1965. His outline concerns the development of disabilities and rehabilitation. In this model, specific assessments and measurements can be placed on a logical pathway into their own categories (Fig. 6.2). In **Nagi's disablement process model**, the consequences of diseases or aging manifest as impairments in organ systems and functional impairments (impairments; e.g., weakening of muscle strength, hearing loss). Impairments in organ systems lead to problems in fundamental human activities. This category is referred to as functional limitations (functional limitations; e.g., walking, climbing stairs, squatting, speaking, grasping with the hand). Impaired abilities in these areas, in turn, predispose individuals to disabilities, which manifest as difficulties or inability to perform essential activities of daily living (disability; e.g., household chores, self-care, hobbies). In this model, functional limitations, which can be assessed through surveys or standardized measurements such as walking speed measurement, form an important link between impairments in organ systems and limitations and disabilities.

In 1994, Lois M. Verbrugge and Alan Jette published an article in which they developed Nagi's disablement model into a **socio-medical disablement model** by adding an environmental dimension (physical, social) and an individual factors dimension (unfavorable or favorable characteristics such as lifestyles, body mass index, psychological characteristics) [36]. Individual factors include lifestyle and

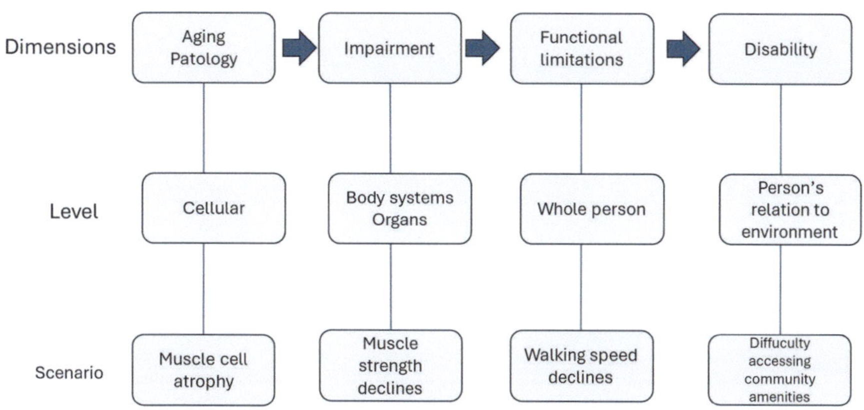

Fig. 6.2 Nagi's disablement process model is presented as dimensions, level of systems and potential scenario of consequences

behavior changes, psychosocial attributes and coping mechanisms, and activity accommodations. Extra-individual factors include medical care and rehabilitation, medications and other therapeutic regimens, external supports, and the built, physical, and social environment. Additionally, it contains risk factors, which are predisposing factors that elevate the chances for functional limitation and disability when chronic conditions occur and progress.

The ecological model of aging or the "competence-press model" by M. Powel Lawton and Lucille Nahemow [17] considers human engagements to stem from the environment where a person lives and how well its requirements and facilitators support their functional capacity. A person possesses a range competency and the environment a range of demands (Fig. 6.3). Personal competence comprises physical and cognitive functioning, skills, abilities, and health. The environment can be outlined as physical environment, and the social environment extending from immediate social milieu to the society at large. Ecology is used in the sense that it emphasizes the interdependence elements in a system on each other. The ecology of aging refers to the adaptation of a person to their environment and the alteration of the environment as part of the process of human adaptation. The aging process itself is seen as the process of continuous adaptation: adaptation to the external environment and to the changes in functional capacity with aging. The ecological model of aging considers that specific combinations of individual competence and environmental

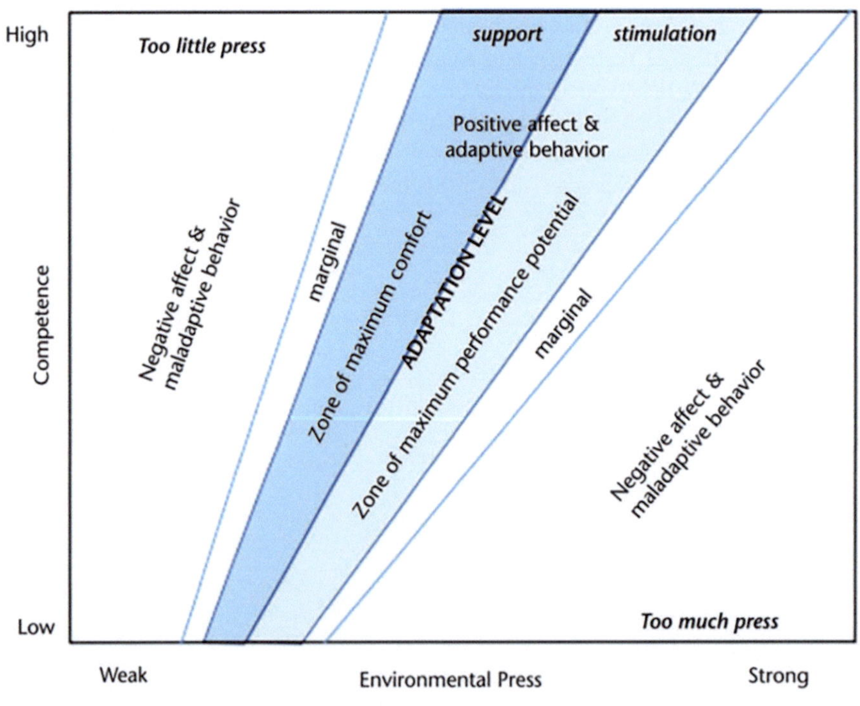

Fig. 6.3 The press-competence model [17]

demands and supports can offer an ideal individualized circumstance for functioning. This is called person-environment (P-E) fit. Persons with declined competence are more susceptible to environmental press than those with higher competence. When environmental press and individual competence match, the result may be adaptative behavior. In case they do not match, the likelihood of maladaptive behavior and diminished well-being increase.

The socioecological model of active living [30] comprises four domains of active living: active transport, occupational activities, household activities, and active recreation. This model successfully incorporated multiple contextual factors relevant for active living into intrapersonal, perceived environment, behavior, physical environment, and policy environment layers, which were visually nested with the individual in the center. For example, the intrapersonal layer includes demographic factors, the perceived environment layer includes subjectively evaluated features of the environment, the behavior settings layer includes objectively features of the environment, and the policy layer comprises issues such as organizing, regulating, and guiding public services and tasks. This model may be used as a framework that provides an outline for other more detailed models of specific active living aspects within its layers. For example, the ecological model of aging proposed by Lawton and Nahemow [17] focuses on the intrapersonal, behavior, and behavior setting layers posited in the social ecological approach.

In 2001, the World Health Organization published the **International Classification of Functioning, Disability and Health (ICF)**, which describes how diseases and disabilities can be related to an individual's life (Fig. 6.4). In the ICF model, health and the individual and environment interact with each other. The ICF model does not present a clear path of decline or improvement in functional

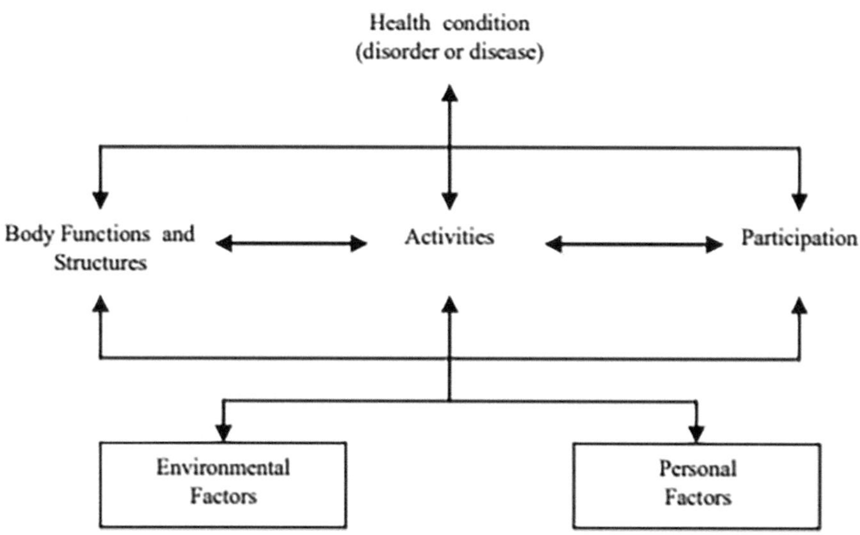

Fig. 6.4 The interactions between the component of ICF [38]

capacity but emphasizes the relationships between different factors. The ICF describes functioning as body structures and functions, activities, and participation in various life situations and community life. Instead of using the term disability, the ICF model uses the term participation in various life situations and community life. Participation and promoting participation opportunities are important goals of support, services, and rehabilitation. Participation opportunities can be improved by modifying the external environment, even if the individual's functional capacity itself does not change. Models focusing on disabilities concentrate more on the individual and see the individual's physical and psychological characteristics as important targets for rehabilitation. In the ICF model, functional impairments are not seen as individual characteristics but rather as a combination of circumstances, many of which stem from the social environment. By altering the environment, it is possible to enable the participation of individuals with functional impairments in various areas of life. In practice, both rehabilitation and support measures targeted at the individual and environmental adaptation and changes are implemented when functional capacity and participation opportunities decline. The main dimensions in the ICF model are presented neutrally so that they encompass both positive and negative dimensions, allowing them to describe both healthy and unhealthy individuals. Table 6.5 lists the main dimensions of participation in the ICF model. The ICF model strongly emphasizes the significance of the environment and society in determining the consequences of disabilities for individuals.

Since 2015 the WHO has started to promote the idea that functional ability consists of the intrinsic capacity of the individual, relevant environmental characteristics and the interaction between them. *Intrinsic capacity* refers to the functioning of an individual independent of the environment and comprises the mental and physical capacities that a person can draw on and can be described as their ability to walk, think, see, hear, and remember. The criticism of the concept of intrinsic capacity has highlighted the unclear measurement model. Even though intrinsic capacity should be a positive construct, most studies are lacking assessments of the positive dimension of functioning and instead they use the absence of deficits—which is merely the reverse side of the deficits [13]. Therefore, thus far most intrinsic capacity studies have failed to generate new knowledge but rather contributed redundant information, because it has been evident for decades that functional deficits predict adverse outcomes. *Vitality capacity* is considered the underlying physiological determinant of intrinsic capacity. A working group of WHO suggested that vitality capacity is a physiological state resulting from the interaction between multiple physiological systems, reflected in the energy metabolism, neuromuscular function, and immune and stress response functions of the body [2]. Vitality capacity is a relatively new concept and has not been established in scientific literature. It seems presumable that this concept can be similarly criticized as the intrinsic capacity.

In 2011, the **National Health and Aging Trends Study** (NHATS) combined features from Nagi's model and the ICF model (Fig. 6.5). The NHATS model has a clear structure for the pathway leading to disabilities. The model includes a category measuring capacity, which corresponds to the category of functional limitations in Nagi's model and has an additional category describing adaptation of function and

Table 6.5 Dimensions on activities and participation in the ICF model [38]

Main dimension	Description	Examples
Learning and applying knowledge	Involves intentional sensory experiences and cognitive functions	Watching, listening, reading, writing, acquiring skills, applying knowledge, solving problems
General tasks and demands	Relates to general aspects of task completion, organization, and management	Organizing daily routines, time management, planning, taking responsibility, handling stress, and crises
Communication	Encompasses understanding and producing verbal and non-verbal messages	Understanding spoken language, using symbols, engaging in conversation, using communication devices
Mobility	Concerns the movement of the body and objects and the use of transportation	Standing, walking, lifting, grasping, moving indoors and outdoors, using transportation
Self-care	Involves activities related to maintaining personal health and hygiene	Washing, dressing, eating, drinking, toileting, caring for the skin and nails, managing diet, maintaining physical health
Domestic life	Includes actions related to managing a household and supporting other household members	Acquiring housing, food, clothing, cleaning the home, performing household repairs, preparing meals, caring for clothing, assisting other household members
Interpersonal interactions and relationships	Focuses on social interactions and relationships in various contexts	Respect, tolerance, physical contact, establishing relationships, communication in work, friendships, and family
Major life areas	Relates to tasks involving education, employment, and financial activities	Applying for jobs, working, maintaining financial independence, engaging in education
Community, social, and civic life	Involves participation in cultural, religious, political, and social activities	Participating in associations, cultural activities, religious practices, political life, and citizenship
Contextual factors	These are environmental factors that influence participation, either promoting or restricting it	Products and technology, natural environment, human-made changes, support and relationships, attitudes, services, systems, and policies

environment (accommodation) [12]. For example, if individuals in a population study report fewer difficulties in activities of daily living (e.g., bathing), but their capacity (ability to squat, bend, grasp with the hand) has not changed, the explanation may lie in favorable changes in the living environment (improved accessibility of bathrooms). Favorable changes in the social or physical environment or practices may also underlie, for example, increased volunteer work, employment, or participation in organizational activities among older people. According to the NHATS model, changes in individual capacity and changes in the environment or practices may explain trends in population functional capacity and participation.

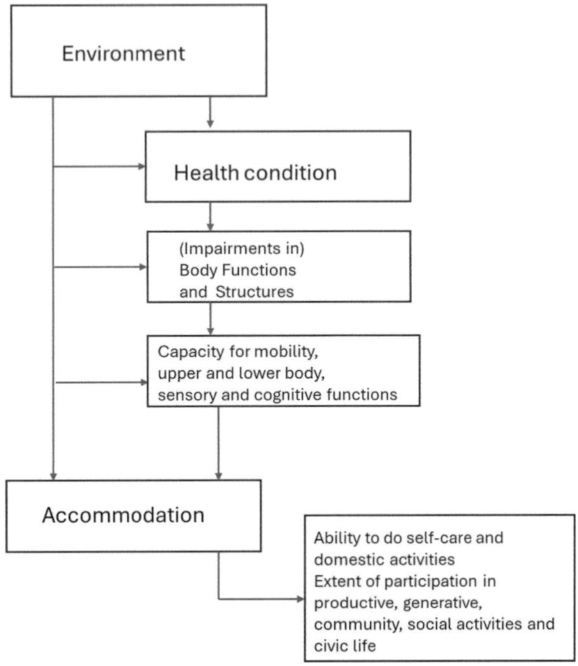

Fig. 6.5 The National Health and Aging Trends Study framework for disability [9]

The NHATS model highlights the ICF term "capacity" to refer to an individual's physiological, cognitive, and sensory capacity to carry out the building blocks of activities (e.g., mobility and other physical movements, learning, remembering, seeing, hearing, and communicating). Such measures are frequently incorporated in Nagi's "functional limitations," whereas the ICF considers these for the most part subdomains of both "activities" and "participation." NHATS envisions assessing these domains mainly through performance measures [9]. A new domain termed accommodations refers to behavioral responses to changes in functional capacity. It includes adaptions such as receiving help, using assistive technology, changes to the environment, and other compensatory strategies such as doing an activity less frequently, more slowly, or differently [37]. In the NHATS model, the ability to carry out self-care (e.g., ADL) and domestic life (e.g., IADL) activities and the extent of participation in productive, generative, community, social, and civic life are considered the outcomes. ADL and IADL reflect what is usually assessed as disability under the Nagi model. The NHATS model explicitly captures also elective and valued activities relevant for quality of life beyond the basics of self-care and domestic life [9]. Participation in elective activities that promote quality of life aligns with the idea of active aging as presented by Rantanen et al. [27].

Table 6.6 summarizes the essential elements of the disablement frameworks described in this chapter.

Table 6.6 A comparison of the elements in the different disablement models

Aspect	Nagi framework	NHATS framework	ICF framework	Ecological model of aging (competence-press model)
Starting point	Pathology	Health conditions and environment	Health conditions and environment	Personal competence and environment
Focus	Impairments and functional limitations as predictors of disability	Task and environmental accommodations as modifiers of the capacity and ability interaction	Interrelationships of body functions and environment	Interaction between individual competence and environmental demands (P-E fit)
Disability definition	Difficulty or inability in ADL and IADL	(in)ability to do essential ADL and IADL and participate in elective activities	Participation in activities and social life	Maladaptive behavior when competence and environment are mismatched
Environment's role	Indirectly mentioned	Accommodations may reduce environmental requirements	Directly influences activities and participation	Central to the model (physical and social environment)
Personal factors	Not explicitly considered	Considered through capacity	Explicit consideration of personal factors	Focused on personal competence and its interaction with the environment
Endpoint	Disability	Ability to carry out essential activities Extent of participation in pleasing and elective activities	Participation in social and civic life	Adaptive or maladaptive behavior depending on person-environment fit

6.5 Preclinical Functional Decline or Adaptive Behavioral Change?

Many older individuals do not report difficulties in performing certain tasks but nonetheless indicate that they have changed their way of doing the task in some way. These changes may include slowing down, using assistive devices, taking breaks during tasks, performing the task less frequently, or ceasing them altogether. A situation in which a person reports changes but does not report difficulties in performing the task is referred to as preclinical functional limitation. This term was launched by Dr. Linda Fried in the 1990s. The idea was that before the person experiences manifest disability, there may be a "preclinical state" that can be identified

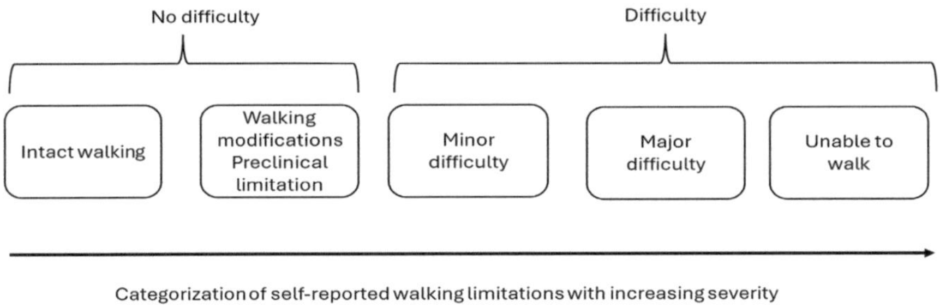

Fig. 6.6 Categorization of walking limitations. The severity progresses from left to right. (Modified from a scheme by [18])

to help targeting interventions [10]. The additional benefit is that ability to classify the heterogeneous group of individuals who report no difficulties, e.g., in walking specific distances, but whose physical capacity may range from top-level masters' athletes to just being able to do the task. In this context, identifying a preclinical state will be a useful tool for predicting disability. Preclinical functional declines were subsequently found to increase the risk of functional limitations in the coming years [11].

Figure 6.6 shows the categorization of self-reported walking limitations with increasing severity. To examine whether the progression of walking decline presented in Fig. 6.6 is valid, we followed up 302 persons aged 75–81 years for 2 years with examinations every 6 months. At baseline, four subgroups were created according to self-reported preclinical mobility limitation in any of the three selected mobility tasks (walking 2 km, walking 0.5 km, climbing stairs): no limitation, preclinical limitation, and minor and major manifest limitation. At baseline, participants with preclinical mobility limitation showed intermediate levels of walking speed and muscle power, compared with those with no limitation or manifest mobility limitation. Participants reporting baseline preclinical mobility limitation had three to six-fold higher age- and sex-adjusted risk of progressing to major manifest mobility limitation during the 2-year follow-up compared with participants with no limitation at baseline, whereas the risk among those with minor limitation at baseline was 14- to 18-fold higher compared with those with no limitation. The self-report assessment tool proved to be a valid measure to capture the early signs of walking limitation and may serve as an inexpensive tool for identifying people without walking limitations who have a high risk for future walking limitations [18].

An alternative way to view changes in doing a task is to consider them as adaptive modifications, by which a person seeks to reduce both the task's demands and the challenges posed by the environment. Doing differently may help older adults continue their valued activities even though early signs of disablement may have emerged. We formed categories based on reported changes or difficulties in walking 2 km as follows: (1) no difficulties and no changes in walking, (2) no difficulties but changes in walking, and (3) difficulties. Life-space mobility was highest among those who reported no difficulties in walking 2 km and lowest among those who reported difficulties. The group that had changed their way of walking was in

Table 6.7 Comparison of two interpretations of the meaning of task modification when predicting functional decline

Aspect	Preclinical disability	Task modification
Studied with questions on	Changes in the way of doing different tasks	Changes in the way of doing different tasks
Meaning	Early sign of disability	Adaptive adjustment made to reduce the burden of activities and environmental requirements
Level of functioning	Intermediate between intact functioning and manifest disability	Intermediate between intact functioning and manifest disability
Interpretation	Predicts disability	An adaptive change that helps maintain opportunities for engagement in important activities when facing functional decline

between these two categories. During a 2-year follow-up, the life-space mobility of those reporting difficulties decreased most sharply and consistently throughout the study period. Those who did not report difficulties at the start of the study maintained their life-space mobility at the highest level. Those who had modified their way to walking 2 km retained their level of mobility within their living environment for the first year of follow-up, with a decline observed only in the second year. Thus, modifying one's approach to activities helped maintain life-space mobility and delayed the reduction of their life-space mobility suggesting sustained access to meaningful destinations [25]. This may help continue hobbies and sustain personally important activities that require leaving home (see Table 6.7).

Changes in ways of doing a task can further be categorized into adaptive (favorable) and maladaptive (unfavorable). Adaptive changes aim to enable continued activity, such as walking, by reducing the task's burden (e.g., slowing down, taking breaks, using assistive devices). Maladaptive changes, on the other hand, are related to reducing or stopping the activity. During the 2-year follow-up, maladaptive changes made to walking 2 km led to a sharper decline in outdoor mobility autonomy compared to no changes or only adaptive changes. This outcome was not explained by differences in lower limb functioning, health, depressive symptoms, memory problems, or socioeconomic status [32, 33].

6.6 Exhausting or Easy?

Greater nuance in self-reporting or test results can be achieved by asking individuals how exhausting or easy they find the task. Reporting fatigue is quite common among older adults. In recent years, fatigue research has expanded within gerontology, as fatigue and susceptibility to fatigue have been found to predict unfavorable health outcomes. Fatigue is an unpleasant symptom that hinders a person's usual performance and can range from mild tiredness to exhaustion. Fatigability is a characteristic related to a specific task with standardized duration and intensity. Fatigue, particularly in relation to muscle load or endurance, has been studied extensively in physiology. Some research has been conducted in gerontology on fatigue during daily activities, and it has been found to increase with age. Fatigue can be categorized into physical, psychological, and emotional fatigue. It may be challenging for individuals to distinguish between these, as a primarily physically exhausting task may also be perceived as psychologically and emotionally tiring. Fatigue can be studied by asking people how exhausting they find various tasks. Another approach is to ask individuals during a specific task (such as during a 6-min walk test) how exhausting they find it at that moment. Slowing down during a task is an adaptive change related to fatigue, potentially due to factors such as reduced aerobic capacity, decreased muscle strength, and the age-related decline in movement efficiency.

6.7 Autonomy in Mobility

Autonomy refers to the perceived freedom to make one's own decisions and to be in charge of one's actions. Autonomy is one of the fundamental psychological needs and an essential element of life satisfaction and engagement in meaningful activities [28]. Autonomy when growing old often may align with functional capacity; however, functional limitations do not necessarily exclude loss of autonomy. Most often autonomy of older adults has been studied in long-term care settings, where advanced functional deficits and high care needs place specific preconditions for satisfying the autonomy needs of residents. Autonomy is a relevant topic for research also among more vigorous and community-living older people.

Autonomy in mobility refers to an individual's satisfaction with their ability to move to destinations of interest and participate in out-of-home activities as they desire. It pertains to the ability to plan and engage in activities outside the home, such as visit relatives and friends, take trips, travel, enjoy leisure time, meet others, and live life as they wish [3]. It is quite common that the transportation needs of older people with mobility impairments are not met [4]. However, in many cases, autonomy in mobility may be sustained also among people with functional limitations by environmental modifications and transportation assistance.

We have launched the concept of unmet physical activity need which stems from a critical appraisal of the feasibility of promoting physical activity among older adults. In our study, many older people wished to increase their physical activity but felt they lacked the opportunity to do so, a situation we termed unmet physical activity need [22]. Unmet physical activity need was more common among those with walking difficulties, depressive symptoms, and musculoskeletal diseases [22]. Additionally, the accumulation of risk factors, including low socioeconomic status, self-reported walking difficulty, and lack of social support, increased the risk of unmet physical activity needs [6]. Unmet physical activity need is distinct from physical inactivity. All people with low physical activity levels do not perceive unmet physical activity need. We found that lower neighborhood mobility and decreased physical activity levels often precede the development of unmet physical activity needs, especially if these declines took place in recent past [19, 22].

6.8 Person-Environment Interaction Underlying Mobility

Outdoor mobility requires not only the physical ability to move independently and safely from one place to another but also the capacity to navigate environmental challenges, such as stairs, uphill paths, or uneven surfaces, and avoid getting lost. Consequently, environmental factors are crucial determinants of mobility in old age. Because older people often engage in activities close to home, the neighborhood environment significantly influences outdoor mobility among older adults. Research on the physical environment and outdoor mobility has primarily focused on examining the associations between the neighborhood environment and total physical activity. In these studies, environmental features have comprised factors such as the availability of services and destinations, pedestrian infrastructure, traffic safety, walkability, residential density, and street connectivity. Some of these environmental features can be directly measured using observational techniques, such as geographic information systems (GIS), while others can only be assessed through individuals' perceptions via self-report instruments. Observational techniques aim to capture information about the actual environment, whereas perceived environmental data is influenced by a person's past experiences, personal capacity, and social factors. The agreement between observational and self-report measures is often low to moderate, highlighting the significant differences in the information they provide.

Environmental factors can either facilitate or hinder outdoor mobility depending on an individual's functional capacity and preferences [29]. People may perceive the same neighborhood and living environment differently. For example, hills in the vicinity may serve as a fitness challenge for some but may hinder walking for older adults [6, 29]. Additionally, a safe, walkable, and aesthetically pleasing neighborhood can positively influence older adults' participation in out-of-home physical activities. Physical activity levels are also higher among older adults who live in areas with favorable pedestrian infrastructure, including the availability of resting places and nearby destinations, such as recreational facilities or parks. To support self-reporting, we have developed a list of environmental features that facilitate walking and those that hinder walking (see Tables 6.8 and 6.9). In our study, those with restricted life-space were less likely to report mobility facilitators in their environment and more likely to report mobility barriers [24].

Perceptions of the environment may either constrain or extend older people's life-space. Environmental facilitators (resting places, even walkways) may compensate for the declined physical capacity and alleviate the strain of walking longer distances by enabling the use of adaptive walking modifications (rest breaks, using an aid), while lack of such facilitators fuels avoidance of walking longer distances [32, 33]. Conversely, environmental demands that exceed a person's capacity are risk factors for the development of walking difficulties over time [14]. Poor street conditions or a lack of resting places, for example, are associated with an increased risk of developing walking difficulties [14, 25]).

Table 6.8 Perceived environmental facilitators for outdoor mobility reported by community living people aged 75–90 who had vs. did not have restricted life-space mobility

	Restricted life-space mobility	
Perceived environmental facilitator outdoors	Yes %	No %
Park or other green area	36.2	43.6
Walking trail, skiing track	43.7	66.8
Nature, lakeside	63.5	79.0
Familiar environment	63	64
Appealing scenery	64	70
Own yard	54	59
Other people outdoors motivate	18	23
Good lighting	30	43
Peaceful and good quality walkways	49	51
Even sidewalks	31	29
Resting places by the walking route	22	19
Walkways without steep hills	12	13
Services close; shops, market, etc.	41	46
No car traffic	11	15
No cyclists on walkways	4	5
Safe crossings: Traffic lights, zebra crossing, or traffic island between lanes	19	27

Table 6.9 Perceived environmental barriers for outdoor mobility reported by community living people aged 75–90 who had vs. did not have restricted life-space mobility

	Restricted life-space	
Perceived environmental barrier outdoors	Yes %	No %
Poor street conditions	23	15
High curbs	14	3
Hills in nearby environment	33	17
Long distances to services	18	8
Lack of benches	23	11
Lack of benches in winter	24	15
Noisy environment	5	3
Busy traffic	11	6
Dangerous crossroads	12	7
Cyclists on walkways	21	18
Snow and ice	63	46
Insecurity due to other pedestrians	7	5
Vehicles on walkways	3	1
Poor lighting	4	3
Lack of sidewalks	4	3

We compared visited activity destinations among older people with varying degrees of walking limitations. On a digital map, participants located physical exercise, attractive, and regular destinations they had visited during the past month. Participants with intact walking reported more physical exercise and attractive destinations than those with walking difficulty, and they also visited destinations further away from home than those with walking difficulty. We observed that people with walking difficulty reported fewer destinations other than regular destinations, e.g., shops or healthcare facilities. It is possible that perceiving walking difficulty leads to abandoning destinations for recreational activities, which in turn decreases the life-space, potentially leading to reduced well-being [35].

References

1. Baker PS, Bodner EV, Allman RM. Measuring life-space mobility in community-dwelling older adults. J Am Geriatr Soc. 2003;51:1610–4.
2. Bautmans I, et al. WHO working definition of vitality capacity for healthy longevity monitoring. Lancet Healthy Longev. 2022;3:e789–96.
3. Cardol M, de Haan RJ, de Jong BA, van den Bos GA, de Groot IJ. Psychometric properties of the impact on participation and autonomy questionnaire. Arch Phys Med Rehabil. 2001;82:210–6.
4. Casado BL, van Vulpen KS, Davis SL. Unmet needs for home and community-based services among frail older Americans and their caregivers. J Aging Health. 2011;23:529–53.
5. Cooper R, Kuh D, Hardy R, Mortality Review Group, FALCon and HALCyon Study Teams. Objectively measured physical capability levels and mortality: systematic review and meta-analysis. BMJ. 2010;341:c4467.
6. Eronen J, von Bonsdorff M, Rantakokko M, Rantanen T. Environmental facilitators for outdoor walking and development of walking difficulty in community-dwelling older adults. Eur J Aging. 2013;11:67–75.
7. Eronen J, von Bonsdorff M, Rantakokko M, et al. Socioeconomic status and life-space mobility in old age. J Aging Phys Act. 2016;24:617–23.
8. Eronen J, Portegijs E, Rantanen T. Health-related resources and social support as enablers of digital device use among older Finns. J Public Health. 2024. https://doi.org/10.1007/s10389-024-02241-y
9. Freedman VA. Adopting the ICF language for studying late-life disability: a field of dreams? J Gerontol A Biol Sci Med Sci. 2009;64:M1172–4.
10. Fried LP, Bandeen-Roche K, Williamson JD, et al. Functional decline in older adults: expanding methods of ascertainment. J Gerontol A Biol Sci Med Sci. 1996;51:M206–14.
11. Fried LP, Bandeen-Roche K, Chaves PH, Johnson BA. Preclinical mobility disability predicts incident mobility disability in older women. J Gerontol A Biol Sci Med Sci. 2000;55:M43–52.
12. Guralnik JM, Patel K, Ferrucci L. Assessing functional status and disability in epidemiological studies. In: Newman AB, Cauley JA, editors. The epidemiology of aging. Dordrecht: Springer; 2012. p. 91–118.
13. Hoogendijk EO, Dent E, Koivunen K. Intrinsic capacity: an under-researched concept in geriatrics. Age Ageing. 2023;52:afad183.
14. Keskinen KE, Rantakokko M, Suomi K, Rantanen T, Portegijs E. Nature as a facilitator for physical activity: Defining relationships between the objective and perceived environment and physical activity among community-dwelling older people. Health Place. 2018;49:111–19. https://doi.org/10.1016/j.healthplace.2017.12.003
15. Kontto J, Paalanen L, Sund R, rt al. Using multiple imputation and intervention-based scenarios to project the mobility of older adults. BMC Geriatr. 2022;9(22):311.

16. Kulmala J, Viljanen A, Sipila S, et al. Poor vision accompanied with other sensory impairments as a predictor of falls in older women. Age Aging. 2009;38:162–7.
17. Lawton MP, Nahemow L. Ecology and the aging process. In: Eisdorfer C, Lawton MP, editors. The psychology of adult development and aging. Washington, DC: American Psychological Association; 1973.
18. Mänty M, Heinonen A, Leinonen R, et al. Construct and predictive validity of a self-reported measure of preclinical mobility limitation. Arch Phys Med Rehabil. 2007;88:1108–13.
19. Palmberg L, Portegijs E, Rantanen T, et al. Neighborhood mobility and unmet physical activity need in old age: a 2-year follow-up. J Aging Phys Act. 2019;28:442–7.
20. Portegijs E, Tsai LT, Rantanen T, Rantakokko M. Moving through life-space areas and objectively measured physical activity of older people. PLoS One. 2015;7(10):e0135308.
21. Pynnönen K, Törmäkangas T, Heikkinen RL, et al. Does social activity decrease risk for institutionalization and mortality in older people? J Gerontol B Psychol Sci Soc Sci. 2012;67:765–74.
22. Rantakokko M, Iwarsson S, Hirvensalo M, et al. Unmet physical activity need in old age. J Am Geriatr Soc. 2010;58:707–12.
23. Rantakokko M, Portegijs E, Viljanen A, et al. Life-space mobility and quality of life in community-dwelling older people. J Am Geriatr Soc. 2013;61:1830–2.
24. Rantakokko M, Iwarsson S, Portegijs E, et al. Associations between environmental characteristics and life-space mobility in community-dwelling older people. J Aging Health. 2015;27:606–21.
25. Rantakokko M, Portegijs E, Viljanen A, Iwarsson S, Rantanen T. Mobility modification alleviates environmental influence on incident mobility difficulty among community-dwelling older people: a two-year follow-up study. PLoS One. 2016;22(11):e0154396.
26. Rantanen T. Promoting mobility in older people. J Prev Med Public Health. 2013;2:S50–4.
27. Rantanen T, Eronen J, Kauppinen M, Kokko K, Sanaslahti S, Kajan N, Portegijs E. Life-space mobility and active aging as factors underlying quality of life among older people before and during COVID-19 lockdown in Finland-a longitudinal study. J Gerontol A Biol Sci Med Sci. 2021;76(3):e60–7. https://doi.org/10.1093/gerona/glaa274.
28. Ryan RM, Deci EL. Self-determination theory and the facilitation of intrinsic motivation, social development, and wellbeing. Am Psychol. 2000;55:68–78.
29. Sakari R, Rantakokko M, Portegijs E, et al. Do associations between perceived environmental and individual characteristics and walking limitations depend on lower extremity performance level? J Aging Health. 2017;29:640–56.
30. Sallis JF, Cervero RB, Ascher W, et al. An ecological approach to creating active living communities. Annu Rev Public Health. 2006;27:297–322.
31. Satariano WA, Guralnik JM, Jackson RJ, et al. Mobility and aging: new directions for public health action. Am J Public Health. 2012;102:1508–15.
32. Skantz H, Rantanen T, Palmberg L. Outdoor mobility and use of adaptive or maladaptive walking modifications among older people. J Gerontol A Biol Sci Med Sci. 2020a;75:806–12.
33. Skantz H, Rantanen T, Rantalainen T, et al. Associations between perceived outdoor environment and walking modifications in community-dwelling older people: a two-year follow-up study. J Aging Health. 2020b;32:1538–51.
34. Tsai LT, Rantakokko M, Viljanen A, et al. Associations between reasons to go outdoors and objectively-measured walking activity in various life-space areas among older people. J Aging Phys Act. 2016;24:85–91.
35. Tuomola EM, Keskinen KE, Rantanen T, Portegijs E. Associations between walking limitations and reported activity destinations among older adults. Eur J Aging. 2024;21:16.
36. Verbrugge LM, Jette AM. The disablement process. Soc Sci Med. 1994;38:1–14.
37. Weiss CO, Hoenig HM, Fried LP. Compensatory strategies used by older adults facing mobility disability. Arch Phys Med Rehabil. 2007;88:1217–20.
38. World Health Organization. International classification of functioning, disability, and health, ICF. Geneva: World Health Organization; 2001.

Promoting Engagement in Meaningful Activities

7

Abstract

Active engagement in meaningful activities means that people conduct voluntary and purposeful actions that have consequences to themselves and to their environment, rather than just having things happening to them. Active engagement in meaningful activities continues even though peoples' capacities and abilities may decline; the activities may just change form. There are many approaches to fostering this scenario, and the measures may take place on different levels of individual's physical, emotional, cognitive, and social functioning, physical and social environment, and policy. Ideally, older people may participate in productive activities such as paid and unpaid work, social life, leisure, intellectual and cultural life, and civic engagement according to their own priorities and capacities.

7.1 An Empirical Model of Active Aging

When developing the model of active aging, we paid attention to not confusing active aging with its determinants or consequences (see Fig. 7.1). We acknowledged that some earlier discussion concerning active aging was tangled in the sense that some tried to define active aging as a state or a phenotype and listed external normative criteria. This resulted in descriptions of elite individuals who were to have characteristics and a life approach unattainable for most. Sometimes correlates or preconditions of active aging have been confused with active aging.

Active aging is an individualized process that depends on the environment and a person's capacities and aspirations, all of which are considered preconditions for active aging. Quality of life is coproduced in the context of the persons own capacities and environmental support and modified by the individual's active aging process. An individual's active aging process refers to their activity that is in line with

T. Rantanen, *Advancing Research on Active Aging and Participation*, https://doi.org/10.1007/978-3-031-94702-5_7

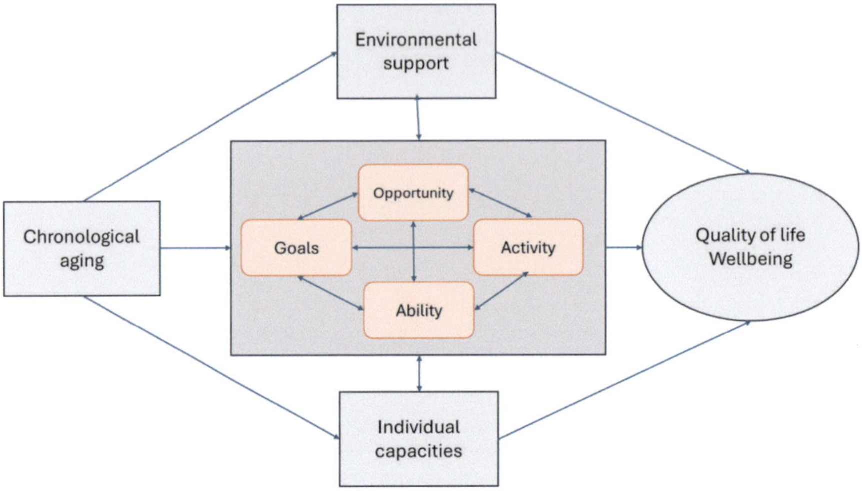

Fig. 7.1 Active aging in an individual's life concerns the dynamics of what activities one wants to do (goals), what activities one can do (ability), autonomy in doing activities (opportunities), and what and how much activities one does (activity). The factors that either support or hinder active aging are environmental support and individual capacities that change with aging. Environmental support may comprise services, environmental modifications, neighborhood features, or social support. The individual capacities include cognition, sensory functioning, muscle strength, and ability to move oneself from one place to another. These are internal capacities of the body that one can draw from when performing activities

their goals, opportunities, and abilities in the context of their life situation. The goals, ability, and opportunity underlie the outcome of active engagement in life situations. Active engagement, in turn, contributes to experiences that underlie quality of life and other elements of well-being. The process of active aging is in line with similar models that have been presented in other fields of study, such as economics, employment research, political science, and research on health behavior change, with all these fields using slightly different terminology in their models that still reflect similar scheme of things. Basically, these models suggest that goals, opportunities, and abilities underlie behavior.

Our model of active aging was inspired by the ecological model of aging, presented by Lawton and Nahemow [5], and the selective optimization with compensation (SOC) model, presented by Baltes and Baltes [2]. The ecological model of aging focuses on the person-environment relationship. In the ecological model, human behavior depends on personal capabilities, competencies, and the living environment. The individual competence in the ecological model refers to a person's functional capacity. In our model, individual capacities describes all capacities that the person has (e.g., muscle strength, vision, cognitive capacity), while abilities relate to skill and abilities to do different tasks, such as use a computer, find information, do DIY, or exercise. The environmental component includes various aspects of the living environment, such as the physical, social, and personal environment.

Based on the ecological model, older people with lower competence are more prone to environmental press, such barriers in the living environment, which will lead to adapting and changing behaviors. In adaptive behavior changes, physical competence and environmental demands are balanced, and the individual can continue carrying out personally valued tasks. In contrast, a situation in which environmental demands exceed individual capacity may lead to maladaptive behaviors, manifested as doing things less often or avoiding some tasks [5]. We acknowledge that adaptation also refers to adapting one's goals or adapting one's environment. Older individuals continuously adapt their behavior owing to changes in their personal competence and the demands of the physical environment, which they may also remodel. Selective optimization with compensation (SOC) model, presented by Baltes and Baltes [5], has a similar perspective. Overall, the SOC model offers a framework for understanding developmental change and resilience throughout the lifespan. According to the SOC model, older people respond to functional losses with three types of adaptive behaviors: selection, optimization, and compensation. Selection refers to doing only the most valued activities and abandoning less important activities; optimization is about learning new ways to do the activities; and compensation is about adding a new element into activity, such as an assistive device, remodeling the home, or moving, to keep on doing the desired activity.

The novelty of our model of active aging is that we incorporated goals, i.e., willingness to act in our model. We describe the meaningful activities based on the purpose of the activity rather than exact quantitative criteria for fulfilling specific standard requirements for each activity. Goals are important from the perspective of active aging as people often act according to their goals, which inspire the strivings for activity and may underlie differences in manifestations of the person-environment relationship among different people. The way people execute an activity may change with increasing age even though the purpose of the activity remains the same. For example, at a younger and in more vigorous life stage, a person may exercise in the nature by hiking long distances, while at older ages a stroll in the neighborhood park may serve the same purpose.

7.2 Personal Goals

Personal goals or life goals refer to life situations that people want to achieve or avoid in the future. They may range from small, daily strivings to lifelong undertakings. Goals direct life course. People may set career goals, physical activity goals, or health goals. From the perspective of participation, autonomy, and active aging, setting, pursuing, or modifying goals are important means of guiding life. People inherently modify and re-evaluate their goals or circumstances when life situations change.

Goals form an essential entity in fostering health and well-being. Goal-setting is a core practice, for example, within rehabilitation. The idea of goal-setting is to motivate participation in rehabilitation and to increase behavior change. Particularly goals that relate to real-life situations, are functional, and have personal meaning will motivate people to strive to improve their functioning following adverse health events. Rehabilitation usually takes place after an injury or medical operation, when there is uncertainty about the future life situation. Therefore, rehabilitation goals need to be specific, measurable, attainable, and realistic, and they need to have a time frame.

Overall life resources will influence goal engagement. We studied personal characteristics and socioeconomic, social, and health resources as factors underlying personal goals among 824 community-dwelling people aged 75–90 years. We elicited personal goals using a revised version of the personal project analysis in a structured interview. The most frequently reported goals were related to health maintenance. People with better health were more likely to report goals related to leisure time, social, and physical activities and less likely to report goals related to recovery of health. Those with poor social resources were at risk for having no personal goals in their lives ([14]; see Table 7.1). These findings inspired us to pursue further analyses on how goal setting strategies influence both mental and physical well-being in old age. We studied two distinct strategies aiming at reducing discrepancies between goals and what is feasible for a person. The first was assimilation, which can be described as tenacious goal pursuit. This refers to people increasing effort in adjusting their current situation in line with personal goals. The second is accommodation, which refers to flexible goal adjustment by disengaging from blocked goals or by downgrading their importance [3]. It is not clear whether persistently pursuing specific goals or flexibly adjusting them in old age is the most beneficial coping strategy in terms of active aging. Some researchers have proposed a more important role for flexibility than tenacity for subjective psychological

Table 7.1 Summary of central aspects of personal goals

Aspect	Description
Definition of goals	Goals are things or states individuals seek to achieve, maintain, or avoid in the future
UJACAS goal inquiry	Goals were enquired by asking how much the person had been wanting to do an activity
The role of goals in old age	In old age, when resources diminish, goals motivate individuals to act despite challenges and focus their energy on positive adaptations. To pursue important goals, individuals need to adapt to the changes in themselves and their lives as they age
Goal realization in old age	Old age can enable the realization of important personal goals, not just adaptation to negative changes and losses. Common goals reported include writing memoirs, learning to play an instrument, and spending time at a summer cottage
Health influence on goal setting	People with better health were more likely to report goals related to leisure time, social, and physical activities
Social resources and goal setting	People with poor social resources were at risk of having no personal goals

well-being. Much less attention has been paid to how tenacity vs. flexibility relates to physical functioning and active engagement especially when facing possible functional limitations in old age. We conducted a cross-sectional analysis among 187 community-dwelling people aged 79–93 years to investigate whether tenacious goal pursuit and flexible goal adjustment influence the association between physical performance and participation in leisure activities [17]. We found that despite low physical performance, highly tenacious people had close to mean level of leisure activity participation. Low tenacity was associated with very little activity especially in outdoor activities and social activities outside home. In another study, we found that older people who persistently pursue their goals, but at the same time are also able to change their goals to correspond to their current resources, perceive better possibilities to participate in activities outside the home and that they move across a wider life-space [15]. In contrast, those showing the lowest tenacity and flexibility in pursuing their goals reported the most constraints in out-of-home mobility. Persistency, especially when combined with flexibility in goal pursuit, appears to help older people to be active in their leisure time.

7.3 Opportunity

Our experience is that older individuals often struggle to distinct opportunity to do something from the ability to do it. Opportunity to do something means that you have a chance to do something. It resonates with autonomy in terms that both executive and decisional autonomy are relevant but also the environment underlies opportunity. The ability to do something refers to whether you can or could perform the task.

Perceiving that one has an opportunity to conduct different meaningful activities has several underlying factors. The concept of affordance stemming from research on human-machine interaction and design may provide an idea about how people perceive opportunities for different activities. Research on affordances is an emerging topic in gerontology with most research coming from studies on aging-in-place and more recently from virtual reality research. There may be a range of possibilities for active engagement in the environment, but a person will engage only with few activities. Affordances refer to the potential for actions individuals perceive when interacting with their environment. Affordances underlie the individual acts and their physical and social environment. For a person who wishes to go for a walk, an attractive path close to home is an affordance in the environment by providing a possibility for a safe walk. However, if this person needs to take care of a sick spouse, the path alone is not an affordance for a walk because caring responsibility overrides the desire to take advantage of the walking path. A visit by a nurse taking over the caring responsibility and the presence of the path will together constitute an affordance.

The environment offers an infinite number of affordances for human activity. A person's intentional activity concerns only a fraction of the range of social and environmental potential. The activity or engagement happens when the individual characteristics and resources and the environmental features match (Kyttä 2003, 2004). Affordances are real but they are not properties of either a person or their environment, but stem from this relationship. Aspects such as perceived or anticipated enjoyment, aesthetics, usefulness, and attitude underlie whether affordances will propel activities and engagement.

7.4 Ability

Ability refers to having a skill or physical and psychological ability to perform an activity. Functional abilities and how they may be categorized and evaluated are discussed in Chap. 6. The ICF provides a useful way to categorize abilities in different domains of meaningful activities and participations. Having an ability or skill is not binary, but there are several degrees to an ability to do something. For example, older individuals' digital device use can be considered a continuum, ranging from non-use to learning to use, possibly encountering some difficulty when using, and fluent use [4].

Important personal skills that are gaining more and more scientific attentions are often called **literacies**. Initially literacy referred to having the skills to read, write, speak, and listen. Nowadays its meanings go beyond that. Literacy is a continuum of learning and proficiency in essential life areas such as social interactions, health, work, and physical activity. It includes work-specific skills and skills related to citizenship. We investigated the role of health literacy in active aging among 948 individuals aged 75–85 years. Active aging scores were higher among those with better health literacy and lower among those with more chronic conditions. Health literacy was a stronger predictor than chronic conditions of active aging, and its predictive value remained statistically significant after adjustment for cognitive capacity, number of depressive symptoms, physical performance, and length of education. We concluded that higher health literacy can enable older persons, including those with multiple chronic conditions, to maintain higher levels of active aging. As more people are projected to live with chronic conditions to older ages, health literacy may help them to cope with illnesses and functional limitations and lead a fulfilling life [4]. Definitions of different literacies currently studied in gerontology can be seen in Table 7.2. Literacies are essential for individuals to navigate modern society effectively, make informed decisions, and engage in their communities.

Table 7.2 Definitions of different literacies

Type of literacy	Definition
Health literacy	Understanding health information, navigating healthcare systems, and making informed health decisions
Social literacy	Skills related to communication, social interaction, and understanding social norms and dynamics
Physical literacy	The ability to engage in physical activities confidently and competently
Economic literacy	Understanding economic principles, personal finance, and the functioning of markets and economies
Digital literacy	The ability to find, evaluate, create, and communicate information using digital technologies
Media literacy	Understanding and critically analyzing media content, including news, advertising, and entertainment
Civic literacy	Understanding civic rights and responsibilities, government processes, and participation in civic activities
Environmental literacy	Knowledge about environmental issues, sustainability, and engaging in actions that contribute to a sustainable future
Cultural literacy	Understanding and appreciating cultural differences, norms, and values in a diverse society
Numeracy	The ability to understand and work with numbers, including basic arithmetic and more complex mathematical concepts

7.5 Activity

Activity refers to everything that people do for enjoyment, responsibility, or obligation. Activity is discussed in more detail in Sect. 5.2. Stemming from the traditional aging research approach, the most studied activities are those that form the necessities of daily life (ADL, IADL, mobility) or health-enhancing activities (physical activity, health habits), but activities that create positive or restorative experiences and that people do for enjoyment have been less studied in gerontology. We consider activity to refer to a wider set of different engagements that may include social and domestic activities, leisure activities, physical and intellectual activities, managing finances, helping others, and aesthetic aspirations and pursuits related to world view.

We defined active aging as the striving for activity according to one's own goals, abilities, and opportunities. To quantify active aging, we used the University of Jyväskylä Active Aging Scale (UJACAS), which includes 17 activities described based on their purpose and formulated to capture the respondent's active role (see Sect. 5.5. for more details of the scale). The UJACAS consists of 17 activities that were identified based on an iterative multiphase process. Table 7.3 presents the proportion on older men and women who report doing the activity at least once a week or at least to some extent (depending on the phrasing of the question).

Table 7.3 The proportion of community-living men and women aged 75–85 years who are doing the activities listed in the UJACAS scale at least once a week or at least to some extent

Activity	Men %	Women %
Managing personal finances	96	53
Promoting matters in own life	94	95
Exercising in the nature	91	81
Maintaining social relationships	90	96
Making one's days interesting	90	96
Making one's home cozy	90	93
Training one's brain	85	88
Keeping fit	81	87
Using a computer	77	64
Helping others	71	66
Crafting, DIY	69	56
Taking care of one's appearance	63	78
Doing things according to one's world view	63	60
Learning to know new people	51	66
Promoting societal matters	48	42
Singing, painting or other art	35	35
Attending events	30	45

7.6 Advancing Active Aging

Earlier research suggests that, for example, social engagement, physical activity, or participation in various community and leisure activities is associated with higher life satisfaction and fewer depressive symptoms. We found that active aging correlates with higher quality of life. Quality of life stems from multifaceted perceptions of how satisfied one is with essential sections of one's life, such as health, social relationships, or living environment, and reflects positive life experiences. Among older people, good quality of life is an important public health goal. Satisfaction with possibilities for participation in valued life situations is one of the key components of quality of life in old age. We assessed quality of life with the short version of the Older People's Quality of Life Questionnaire (OPQOL-brief). The scale includes 13 items. They cover a person's satisfaction with life overall, prospects, health, social relationships, activity, leisure, home, safety, and financial situation. Response options range from 1 (strongly disagree) to 5 (strongly agree) and the sum score from 13 to 65, with higher scores indicating higher quality of life. In the current study, the association with the active aging score and quality of life score was high. This is logical and highlights the importance of people's activity of choice as a factor underlying their quality of life [12].

Quality of life describes a person's satisfaction in various aspects of life. Many of these aspects are, at least to some extent, results of one's own efforts, for example, the home, the financial situation, social relationships, and having interesting things to do. The UJACAS enquires a person's will, ability, opportunity, and volume of the efforts to advance these matters, while quality of life assesses how satisfied the person is with the result. Some of the items in the OPQOL and UJACAS scales are in line, but they do not overlap, because they capture different phases of the active aging process in individuals' lives. UJACAS item assesses the active agency in advancing a section of life and an OPQOL item the level of satisfaction with it. We have conducted longitudinal reciprocal analyses on the association of active aging score and quality of life score and found that active aging propels quality of life and not vice versa.

There are several intervention studies among older adults that have focused on behavioral changes in terms of increasing physical activity, adopting cognitive training, promoting balanced nutrition, stepping up social participation, and augmenting coping styles, which have resulted in positive changes in activity and health outcomes, such as perceived memory, emotional balance, self-efficacy, and overall quality of life.

We took a more comprehensive approach by focusing on self-selected activities since active aging manifests in various forms. We presumed that individualized counseling interventions could be a viable method to promote active aging. Counseling involves an interactive process that helps participants gain clearer insights and consider different perspectives about their situation. In this study, the goal was to increase awareness of meaningful and desirable activities likely to yield personal benefits, set new self-selected activity goals, promote autonomous motivation, and support positive changes in activity [10]. We chose a counseling approach that integrates two socio-cognitive theoretical models: self-determination theory [13] and the theory of planned behavior [1]. Self-determination theory addresses motivation as an intrinsic predisposition to engage in positive behaviors, explaining the underlying motivation for everyday activities in older adults. The theory of planned behavior links beliefs with behavior and elucidates how individuals intend to act. When we did the study, there were no previous studies on counseling interventions based on the integrated model. The aim of this 12-month randomized controlled trial was to investigate the effects of the individualized counseling intervention on the UJACAS total score. The intervention group received individually tailored counseling supporting autonomous motivation for active life (one face-to-face session, four phone calls and supportive written material), and the control group received written health information. Participants were community-dwelling men and women aged 75 or 80 years with intermediate mobility function and without cognitive impairment.

The UJACAS total score increased in the intervention group slightly more than in the control group (net benefit 2%), and the increase in the total score was mostly driven by an increase in the activity subscore, while other subscores did not really change [16].

We then examined further which elements of the integrated health behavior change model might explain the changes in activity. We observed that the baseline attitude and change in attitude directly explained the change in the extent of activity. Moreover, autonomous motivation contributed toward increased activity. Our analyses highlighted autonomous motivation and attitudes as influential change constructs [9]. We concluded that it may be possible to promote active aging with individualized counseling, supporting autonomous motivation, but the effect is modest. That was somewhat disappointing and led us to consider whether behavior change interventions among older people need to be more specific and target pre-specified behavioral changes for people expressing an interest in that specific change.

7.7 COVID-19 Pandemic and Active Aging

In academic research, it is rarely possible on a large scale to modify the environmental features and policies underlying active aging. However, such an opportunity presented itself to us in the form of policies placed to control for the spread of the COVID-19 pandemic. As we had population-based data on active aging originating from 2017 to 2018, we wanted to take the opportunity to study how the participants' active aging and other relevant outcomes might change.

In spring 2020, social distancing measures were recommended in Finland for individuals aged 70 and older to prevent the spread of the SARS-CoV-2 virus, which causes COVID-19. Social distancing involved limiting close contact with people outside one's household and avoiding public places. The social distancing was further reinforced by the closure of restaurants, the suspension of physical activity and cultural classes, the shutting down of venues, and the banning of events and gatherings with more than 10 people. As a result, social distancing effectively prevented participation in most activities outside the home that involved other people. In essence, we were able to evaluate what happened when environmental support for active aging was abruptly withdrawn because of various measures taken to restrain the spread of the virus. For research, too, in-person contact was out of question, so all data were collected with mailed questionnaires. Altogether 809 community-living participants initially aged 75, 80, or 85 years at the AGNES study baseline conducted in 2017–2018 took part in the AGNES-COVID-19 survey in May and June 2020.

Of our community-living participants aged 77–87 years, a minority (11%) did not perceive social distancing to have limited their possibility for activities of choice, while 89% of the respondents reported perceiving at least little restrictions, and 24% a great deal of restrictions. We observed that compared to 2 years before, life-space mobility, active aging score, and quality of life declined during the first wave of the pandemic in spring 2020. The active aging score decreased on average 24 points and the life-space mobility score on average 11 points (adjusted for age and sex). These changes were meaningful. For instance, a decline of 10 points in the life-space mobility score corresponds to a reduction in the frequency of trips to town from 4 to 6 times a week to less than once a week. Also, the quality-of-life score declined from 2017–2018 to 2020 [12].

We then wanted to examine whether people with mobility difficulties were more prone to losses in active aging, life-space mobility, and autonomy in outdoor mobility than others. Self-reported walking difficulties over a 2 km distance were categorized into no difficulty, difficulty, and unable to walk. The total UJACAS score declined 24.9 points (SD 23.5) among those without walking difficulty, 27.0 (SD 25.0) among those reporting walking difficulty, and 19.5 (SD 31.2) among those unable to walk 2 km. When adjusted for baseline UJACAS score, those unable to walk 2 km demonstrated the greatest decline. However, self-rated resilience (believing in own ability to pin setbacks) moderated this association: higher self-rated resilience was associated with less declines in active aging scores among persons with or without walking difficulty and with more declines among persons unable to walk 2 km. In a situation when opportunities for leading an active life were compromised, those with less physical and psychological resources become particularly vulnerable to further declines in activity [16].

The profile of activities differed in 2017–2018 at the baseline of the study between those who had mobility difficulties and those without difficulties. In addition, the changes were different for people with and without mobility limitations. Some item scores on opportunity to act and extent of doing an activity, e.g., for making days more interesting and advancing matters according to one's faith or worldview, were better retained amid COVID-19 by those with limited mobility, attenuating group differences [8]. We concluded that even though active aging scores were somewhat compromised in individuals with limited neighborhood mobility, their opportunities for and engagement in several activities not requiring to leave home seemed to be better retained amid COVID-19 than the activities of those with higher baseline life-space mobility. Thus, active aging may be possible despite mobility restriction.

We have subsequently continued following up the changes in life-space mobility and autonomy in outdoor mobility. Of the earlier participants, 657 took part in the third study wave in 2021–2022. At this time, vaccination coverage was high, and most of the restrictions had been lifted. The life-space mobility and autonomy in outdoor mobility partially recovered at the third study wave compared to the second but did not reach the baseline level. People who were not driving a car and those with impaired lower extremity performance had a 2.4- to 3.6-fold adjusted risk of developing restricted life-space mobility over the follow-up period compared to drivers with intact lower extremity performance. For older people, the recovery of community mobility was incomplete after the restrictions stemming from the pandemic were lifted [7]. Older adults with impaired lower extremity performance and who did not drive were particularly vulnerable to developing restricted life-space mobility, a situation that could lead to social isolation and reduced well-being.

The individualized counseling intervention results and the changes observed during the first wave of the COVID-19 pandemic allowed us to compare different measures in promoting active aging. In the presence of environmental support for active aging, the intervention supporting autonomous motivation and enhancing knowledge about the available opportunities for engagement in meaningful activities may foster active aging to some extent. However, withdrawing environmental support for active aging will have a drastic effect on lowering active aging. This suggests that environmental support is a significant enabler of active aging by offering affordances for preferred activities. We also found that some people replaced blocked activities with available activities. This was evident especially for physical activity. We found that total weekly minutes of walking and vigorous physical activity increased especially among people with higher baseline physical performance, while participation in other activities decreased [6].

References

1. Ajzen I. The theory of planned behavior. Organ Behav Hum Decis Process. 1991;50:179–211.
2. Baltes PB, Baltes MM. Psychological perspectives on successful aging: the model of selective optimization with compensation. In: Baltes PB, Baltes MM, editors. Successful aging: Perspectives from the behavioral sciences. New York: Cambridge University Press; 1990. p. 1–34.
3. Brandtstädter J, Renner G. Tenacious goal pursuit and flexible goal adjustment: explication and age-related analysis of assimilative and accommodative strategies of coping. Psychol Aging. 1990;5:58–67.
4. Eronen J, Paakkari L, Portegijs E, et al. Health literacy supports active aging. Prev Med. 2021;143:106330.
5. Lawton MP, Nahemow L. Ecology and the aging process. In: Eisdorfer C, Lawton MP, editors. The psychology of adult development and aging. Washington, DC: American Psychological Association; 1973. p. 619–674.
6. Lindeman K, Karavirta L, Eronen J, et al. Physical activity changes from before to during the first wave of the COVID-19 pandemic among community-dwelling older adults in Finland. J Aging Phys Act. 2023;32:198–206.
7. Lindeman K, Karavirta L, Koivunen K, Keskinen KE, Eronen J, Portegijs E, Rantanen T. Longitudinal changes in life-space mobility and autonomy in participation outdoors among Finnish community-dwelling older adults from pre-COVID-19 to through the pandemic. Aging Clin Exp Res. 2024;36:85.
8. Portegijs E, Keskinen KE, Tuomola EM, et al. Older adults' activity destinations before and during COVID-19 restrictions: from a variety of activities to mostly physical exercise close to home. Health Place. 2021;68:102533.
9. Pynnönen K, Hassandra M, Tolvanen A, et al. Do the integrated theories of self-determination and planned behavior explain the change in active life engagement following a motivational counseling intervention among older people? Soc Sci Med. 2023;339:116409.
10. Rantanen T, Pynnönen K, Saajanaho M, et al. Individualized counselling for active aging: protocol of a single-blinded, randomized controlled trial among older people (the AGNES intervention study). BMC Geriatr. 2019;19:5.
11. Rantanen T, Hassandra M, Pynnönen K, et al. The effect of individualized, theory-based counselling intervention on active aging and quality of life among older people (the AGNES intervention study). Aging Clin Exp Res. 2020;32:2081–90.
12. Rantanen T, Eronen J, Kauppinen M, et al. Life-space mobility and active aging as factors underlying quality of life among older people before and during COVID-19 lockdown in Finland – a longitudinal study. J Gerontol Med Sci. 2021;76:e60–7.
13. Ryan RM, Deci EL. Self-determination theory and the facilitation of intrinsic motivation, social development, and wellbeing. Am Psychol. 2000;55:68–78.
14. Saajanaho M, Rantakokko M, Portegijs E, et al. Life resources and personal goals in old age. Eur J Aging. 2016;133:195–208.
15. Siltanen S, Rantanen T, Portegijs E, et al. Association of tenacious goal pursuit and flexible goal adjustment with out-of-home mobility among community-dwelling older people. Aging Clin Exp Res. 2019;31:1249–56.
16. Siltanen S, Portegijs E, Saajanaho M, et al. Self-rated resilience and mobility limitations as predictors of change in active aging during COVID-19 restrictions in Finland: a longitudinal study. Eur J Ageing. 2021;19:475–84.
17. Tourunen A, Siltanen S, Portegijs, et al. Assimilative and accommodative coping and older people's leisure activities. J Aging Health. 2020;32:778–86.

Further Reading

Bowling A, Hankins M, Windle G, Bilotta C, Grant R. A short measure of quality of life in older age: the performance of the brief Older People's Quality of Life questionnaire (OPQOL-brief). Arch Gerontol Geriatr. 2013;56:181–7.

Fostering Functional Capacity

8

Abstract

Fostering functional capacity comprises promotion of functioning, prevention of functional decline, rehabilitation of functional losses, and compensation for functional deficiencies. The levels of functioning include organ level, person level, and person-environment relationship, which also comprises participation in different life situations. The functional levels are useful to consider for disablement as well as for re-ablement and in the context of rehabilitation. The functioning of organs, such as muscles, changes with increasing age; however, resistance training can counteract age-related decline. With increasing age, deficits may occur in multiple systems requiring more complex approached in restoring functioning. Finally, it may become necessary to employ compensatory strategies.

8.1 Assessment of Physical Functioning

Physical functioning refers to a persons' physical ability to manage daily tasks that are important to them and to move from one position to another. Key physiological characteristics for physical functioning include muscle strength and endurance, cardiovascular fitness, joint function, and control of body posture and movements. Sensory functions such as vision and hearing are also often considered part of physical functioning. For example, the effects of a stroke and subsequent interventions to support recovery can manifest on all four levels of a person's functional capacity. Following a stroke, muscle strength and standing balance may deteriorate, resulting in walking asymmetry and reduced walking speed. Consequently, the person with stroke experiences difficulties moving outdoors and using public transport and may have to give up choir activities as standing while singing feels unsafe and the bus trip is too demanding. Correspondingly, with rehabilitation and compensation,

T. Rantanen, *Advancing Research on Active Aging and Participation*, https://doi.org/10.1007/978-3-031-94702-5_8

functioning of all four levels can be remedied. The strength and balance will bounce back, walking asymmetry is alleviated, and the time they can stand safely increases; a singing buddy will pick them up by a car to the choir practice, where a chair is provided in case they need to rest while singing.

Functional capacity can be classified into four levels:

1. The functioning of organ systems (*impairment*, e.g., vision, hearing, muscle strength).
2. The person ability to meet task demands (*functional limitation*, e.g., slowing of walking speed, instability when standing up from a seated position).
3. The person's ability to meet environmental demands (*disability*, e.g., difficulty in dressing, shopping, handling bank affairs).
4. Participation in meaningful activities (*participation restriction*, e.g., restraints in volunteering, singing in a choir, civil society activities).

Examples of commonly used functional capacity assessment methods in gerontology are described in Table 8.1.

Table 8.1 Examples of assessments of functional capacity often used in aging research

Functional capacity	Assessment	Why it is assessed and what the result indicates
Organ level impairments in functioning		
Muscle strength	Hand grip strength knee extension strength Measured with a dynamometer, aiming to achieve the best possible result	Maximum strength—measuring knee extension strength reflects the muscle strength required for many movements, such as standing up, climbing stairs Hand grip strength is easy to measure and correlates with the strength of other muscle groups Muscle strength measurements are suitable for participants of all fitness levels Muscle mass and nervous system function determine muscle strength Low values predict functional limitations, decline in health, and mortality Recovery from illness, improving nutritional status, and strength training increase muscle strength Simply training grip strength does not significantly improve health or functional capacity otherwise

(continued)

Table 8.1 (continued)

Functional capacity	Assessment	Why it is assessed and what the result indicates
Functional limitations/difficulty meeting task demands		
Walking ability	Self-reports of the degree of difficulty walking specific distances Timing of walks of different lengths, e.g., 10 m, 400 m at usual or maximum pace, distance covered in a specific time (e.g., 6 min.) Distance/time = velocity	Walking ability contributes to the smooth functioning of everyday life Simple assessments for clinical studies and surveys The measurements suit almost all fitness levels, if assistive devices are allowed; surveys suit everyone Slow walking speed and walking difficulty predict decline in mobility and functional capacity, need for assistance, mortality Exercise training maintains and improves walking ability
Postural control and fear of falling	Measurement of sway in different positions, reach test, balance tests incorporating increasingly challenging movements, self-assessment of balance confidence	Postural control is the foundation of all bodily movements The interaction of senses, the nervous system, and the musculoskeletal system determines it. The test is chosen according to the individual's fitness level, ensuring safety during testing is crucial Poor balance and fear of falling predict falls, injuries, and decline in mobility Rehabilitation involves challenging exercises to improve postural control systems
Disability/difficulty meeting environmental demands		
ADL	Questionnaires, observations, nurse's assessment, interview, proxy interview	Describes a person's ability to perform self-care tasks Suitable for assessing patients or individuals with significantly impaired functional capacity, reflects the level of care required Difficulties in activities of daily living (ADLs) indicate a significant and multifactorial decline in functional capacity A rehabilitative approach, occupational therapy, and physical therapy maintain ADL functional capacity
Participation restriction/restraints in engaging in meaningful activities		
Social and productive activities, leisure, artistic activities	Questionnaires, observations, interview, proxy interview	Describe a person's social roles Offer opportunities to promote well-being of self and others Describe social resources

8.2 Changes in Physical Functioning

Muscle strength is defined as the maximal capacity of a muscle, or group of muscles, to exert a force under a given set of conditions. The muscle strength tests are used to identify force production capacity of the muscles, muscle weakness, or to detect changes in muscle strength, e.g., following a training intervention. The strength of specific muscle groups can be tested using standard dynamometers. The muscle contraction may be isomeric (no joint movement) or dynamic (joint moves). Muscle strength is most often measured in terms of voluntary maximum which refers to the highest effort that the person is willing to produce. This and the fact that force production depends on joint angle and the length of the lever arm make it difficult to come up with universal cutoffs for good, adequate, or weak strength beyond specific equipment and protocol used. Consequently, strength test results obtained using different assessment methods or strength levels reported in different studies may not be directly comparable.

The most obvious function of muscles concerns producing voluntary movement through contraction of muscle cells. Thus, muscle function lays the grounds for mobility and most forms of activity. It has long been known that with increasing age, the movement patterns of individuals change, which is one of the most visible changes that happen with age. Cross-sectional studies show that muscle strength reaches its peak around the age of 30 years. If there are no significant changes in health and physical activity, it remains relatively unchanged until around the age of 50. After this, muscle strength begins to decline at an annual rate of about 1%. Due to hormonal changes associated with menopause, women's muscle strength likely weakens more and faster than men's around that age. As age increases, the decline in muscle strength accelerates. After the age of 65, it decreases by about 1.5–2% per year.

The amount of muscle tissue decreases as a person ages, and at the same time the lost muscle tissue is at least partially replaced by fat tissue. According to one study, only 50% of the cross-sectional area of the knee extensor muscle in older people was composed of muscle tissue, with the rest being fat and connective tissue. The decrease in muscle mass is due to the reduction in the number of muscle fibers because of irreversible cell damage or motor neuron death. Age-related muscle mass reduction is driven by the decrease in motor neurons. There are many other mechanisms behind the reduction in muscle mass, such as the decline in hormone levels (estrogens, androgens, growth hormone), insulin resistance associated with increased fat, and behavioral changes such as reduced physical activity and decreased protein intake due to loss of appetite. Inflammatory reactions associated with many diseases are also considered a factor in muscle mass reduction. Additionally, the low-intensity inflammatory state associated with aging (elevated serum C-reactive protein and interleukin-6 concentrations) is linked to the decline in muscle strength. The decrease in muscle mass, muscle weakness, and reduced metabolic reserve are important factors behind functional impairments and increased mortality risk. Cross-sectionally, lower muscle strength was associated with lower muscle mass; however, the changes in muscle strength and mass do not correlate fully. In fact, strength decline may be driven mostly by other factors than loss of mass, such as changes in neural function [2, 11].

When same people are followed over time, a more varied picture is formed about muscle strength changes, which are happening to all directions. Extensive interindividual variation in changes is evident. Using data from approximately 3000 people aged 71–96 years with approximate length of follow-up being 3 years, we found that 22% increased or maintained their baseline strength level, while others showed some decline. Similar findings have been made by other researchers. Those who had lower strength at baseline more likely improved their strength test results over the follow-up period. This demonstrates that changes in old age do not follow a steady pattern from year to year but instead there are fluctuations following from episodes of adverse events, treatments, and subsequent recovery (see Fig. 8.1). However, when followed over longer periods of time, in our study of 27 years, the predominant direction of change is decline. The average annualized strength change was −1.0%. Steeper decline (>1.5%/year) was associated with older age at baseline, greater weight decrease, and chronic conditions such as stroke, diabetes, arthritis, coronary heart disease, and chronic obstructive pulmonary disease. Even though thc average strength decline, grip strength was quite stable. This means that those who had greater grip strength at the baseline also had greater grip strength at the follow-up.

Research on changes in muscle with increasing age was rather limited up until strength training began to gain significant interest among geriatricians and the general population of older people in the 1980s and 1990s. In the late 1980s, researchers with background in geriatrics, nutritional science, and physical

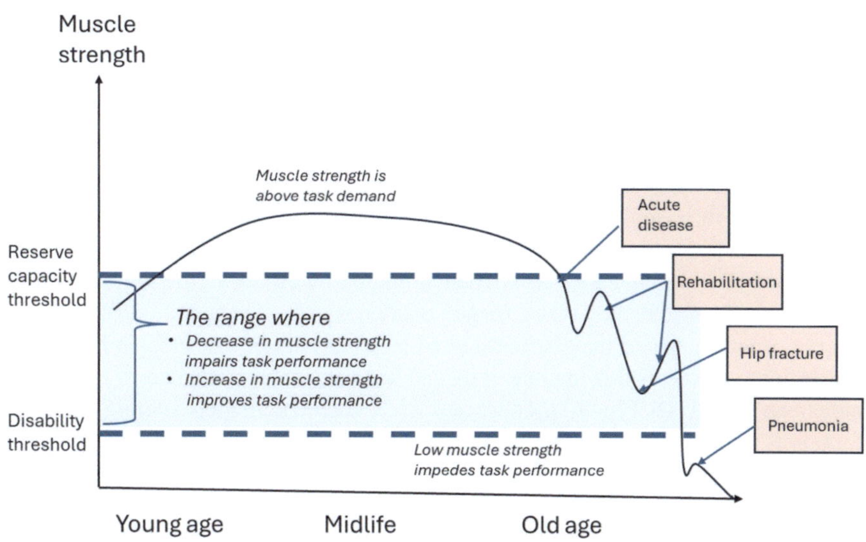

Fig. 8.1 Schematic picture of strength changes across lifespan relative to a theoretical physical task demand

rehabilitation became increasingly interested in muscle changes. This increase in research interest was driven by promising research about the benefits of strength training for older adults demonstrating that older adults could safely engage in strength training and attain improvements in muscle strength and functional ability. The study by Dr. Maria Fiatarone and colleagues in 1990 showed that even nonagenarian and frail individuals could gain muscle mass and strength through resistance training [7]. This study and others like it challenged the previously held belief that age-related muscle loss and weakness were inevitable and irreversible and raised awareness about the importance of physical training and nutrition in restoring muscle functioning. Subsequently, strength training was incorporated into geriatric care and guidelines. Organizations such as the American College of Sports Medicine (ACSM) and the National Institute on Aging began to recommend strength training as a key component of exercise programs for older adults.

Professor Irwin Rosenberg first proposed in 1989 the term sarcopenia to describe the progressive loss of skeletal muscle mass with age. He expected that terming muscle loss as sarcopenia would facilitate interest in the phenomenon, similarly as the term osteoporosis had done for bone research. Since then, the definition of sarcopenia has evolved, and increasing scientific interest has been directed to the research of muscle and aging. In 2016, sarcopenia was added to the International Classification of Diseases with its ICD-10-MC diagnostic code. In 2020 the Sarcopenia Definitions and Outcomes Consortium centered the definition for muscle strength and function [1]. The panel agreed that both muscle weakness defined by low grip strength and slowness defined by low usual gait speed should be included in the definition of sarcopenia. Already earlier consensus articles had shifted focus from muscle mass loss to including also muscle strength loss. This has at least partly been motivated by the aim to find assessment methods and cut points for these assessments that would be feasible and possess optimal translational potential to clinical use.

The importance of muscle strength in physical functions in old age has been established in many studies. The association of muscle strength and functional limitations such as walking speed is strong but not linear. A certain minimum level of muscle strength is needed to do specific physical tasks, such as climbing stairs or opening jars. Below this minimum strength threshold level, people are unable to do the task. A reserve capacity exists when strength is well above the required minimum level. This indicates that strength is adequate for the tasks, and there is a reserve capacity, which may be considered a safety margin that helps prevent disability, for example, following inactivity and deconditioning associated with an episode of an illness (see Fig. 8.1). There have been several attempts to define universal cut points for sarcopenia, but thus far this has not been entirely successful. Strength tests require voluntary effort from the participants, which is challenging to standardize especially in clinical settings. The willingness of participants who are unwell to produce maximum effort may be limited by pain or fear of injury due to exertion. In addition, differences in joint positions during the test and equipment used add to the variation in results.

The concept of reserve of strength as a factor protecting from future disability has been addressed in several studies. One of the first with long follow-up observed that higher handgrip strength measured during mid-life protects from old age functional limitations and disability in initially healthy men [26–28]. The participants were 6089 healthy 45–68-years-old men whose maximal handgrip strength was measured at baseline, and of them, 3218 survivors participated in the disability assessment 25 years after the baseline. Functional limitations included slow customary walking speed ($\leq$0.4 m/s) and inability to rise from a seated position without using the arms. Multiple self-reported upper extremity, mobility, and self-care disability outcomes were also assessed. The risk of disability was more than two times greater in the lowest vs. the highest grip strength tertile. This study showed that middle-aged men with higher handgrip strength were protected from old age disabilities regardless of the diseases that developed over the 25-year follow-up. The higher the reserve capacity in strength is, the less likely people with reach a critical threshold of strength for essential daily movements, such as standing up from a chair or climbing stairs.

In 2021, an umbrella review of systematic reviews and meta-analysis of observational studies on handgrip strength and all health outcomes concluded that grip strength is a useful indicator for general health status, early all-cause mortality, cardiovascular mortality, disability, and leg power assessed as chair rise performance [33]. This also indicates the expansion of research in this area.

8.3 Using Disability Models to Understand Disablement

In the theoretical disablement models, intuitive causal chain emerges; pathology leads to lower muscle strength, which will propel difficulties doing daily tasks. Perceived difficulty doing different tasks will expose to avoiding the tasks subsequently lowering physical activity. This may lead to a vicious circle leading to further decline in strength and worsening of disability [26–28]. The links described here have been well documented in scientific literature. Increased physical activity correlates with greater muscle strength, and greater muscle strength correlates with absence of self-reported mobility difficulties. However, the association of strength with motor performance like walking speed is nonlinear and includes thresholds. Below a certain minimum level of strength, people cannot walk at a given speed [24, 25]. When strength is well above the minimum required level, a reserve capacity exists. At these higher levels, strength increase does not correspond to an increase in walking speed. Being only slightly above the minimum threshold means that almost maximal strength capacity is used when, for example, climbing stairs. This causes discomfort, such as tiredness, and may predispose people to decrease task activity to the minimum essential.

However, in addition to muscle strength, postural control has an essential role in maintaining the ability to walk safely. Minimum levels of lower-extremity strength and the ability to maintain postural stability in the upright position are prerequisites for walking. Better postural balance and lower extremity strength correlate with measured and self-reported walking ability in older persons. In addition, good balance and good muscle strength protect from new disability. In a 4-year prospective study on incident mobility disability, 15.4% of those who were able to hold a full tandem stand for 10 s developed mobility disability, whereas 31.2% of those who were able to hold only a side-by-side stand for 10 s became mobility disabled [23].

Because most studies have focused on independent effects of various impairments, less information is available on risk of disability that results from the combined effects of multiple impairments, termed here co-impairments. It is likely that a decline in function may be better explained by the accumulation of deficits across multiple domains rather than by any single specific impairment. It is possible that people who have a deficit in only one physiological system may be able to compensate for it if they have good capacity in another physiological system. With increasing age, the proportion of those having impairments in multiple physiological systems increases. To develop prevention and rehabilitation programs aimed at decreasing severe walking disability, risk factors for incident walking disability need to be understood.

We conceptualized severe walking disability as inability to walk longer distances and having substantial difficulty in walking even very short distances, evidenced by a very slow walking speed or being unable to walk even minimally. For this study, severe walking disability was defined as being unable to walk or having usual walking speed in the 4-m walk of 0.4 m/second or less and self-reported inability to walk a quarter of a mile. Altogether 758 women who were not severely walking disabled at baseline took part in a 3-year prospective study with six semiannual follow-up data collection rounds following the baseline. Over the course of the study, 173 women became severely disabled in walking. The cumulative incidence of severe walking disability from the first to the sixth follow-up was 7.8%, 12.0%, 15.1% 19.5% 21.2%, and 22.8%. Strength and balance were significant predictors of new walking disability. The relative risk of incident severe walking disability adjusted for age, height, weight, and race was more than five times greater in the group with poorest balance and strength compared with the group with best balance and strength [23]. In addition to poor strength and balance, also other factors contribute to increased risk of walking disability. Obesity combined with low muscle strength increases the risk of decline in walking speed and developing mobility disability, especially among persons <80 years old [34]. Sensory deficits, such as poor vision and hearing, may increase the risk of mobility decline. Older people who have several coexisting sensory difficulties combined with fear of falling are particularly vulnerable to mobility decline. Avoidance of walking as a result of fear of falling is likely to be reinforced when multiple sensory difficulties hinder reception of accurate information about the environment, resulting in accelerated decline in walking ability [39].

These results suggest that the risk of walking disability could be substantially reduced by interventions targeting multiple impairments.

8.4 Co-impairments, Different Training Modalities, and Multicomponent Training

To develop prevention and rehabilitation programs aimed at decreasing disability, the risks brought about by different combinations of functional deficits need to be understood. This chapter will concentrate on strength and postural balance. These two functional deficits respond to specific training, while their combined risk may exceed the risk sum of individual deficits.

Principles of strength training also called resistance training can be applied also for the training of older people. Strength training involves exercises designed to improve muscle strength and endurance. Principles of designing safe and effective strength training programs for older people are presented in Table 8.2.

One of the most common functional deficits in old age is often related to balance control. Balance control involves many underlying systems. Biomechanical constraints including muscle weakness in lower extremities and hip, and flexed postural alignment limits the ability to take compensatory steps for postural recovery after a trip. The limit of stability refers to how far the body's center of mass can be moved over its base of support before balance is lost. Anticipatory postural adjustments prior to voluntary movements guarantee stability during step initiation or during rapid arm movements while standing. Automatic postural responses help correct balance after trips or pushes. Sensory integration involves the vestibular system with other sensory when the support surface or visual environments are moving. Dynamic balance during gait is a result of coordination locomotor and sensorimotor

Table 8.2 Principles for designing safe and effective training programs for older people

Principle	Description
Overload	Muscles must be challenged with a load greater than usual to improve strength and performance
Progression	Gradual increase in overload over time to continue making gains in strength and muscle mass
Specificity	Training adaptations are specific to the muscles and type of activity performed
Variation	Incorporating variety to prevent plateaus and reduce the risk of overuse injuries
Individualization	Programs should meet the unique needs, goals, and abilities of everyone
Reversibility	Gains can be lost if the training stimulus is removed; regular training is necessary to maintain benefits
Recovery	Adequate rest and recovery are crucial for muscle repair and growth
Balance	Includes exercises for all major muscle groups to prevent imbalances and injuries
Adaptation	The body adapts to the stress placed on it over time, leading to increased strength and muscle mass
Technique and safety	Proper form and technique are essential to maximize effectiveness and minimize injury risk

Fig. 8.2 A summary of systems underlying maintaining balance. (Modified from [10])

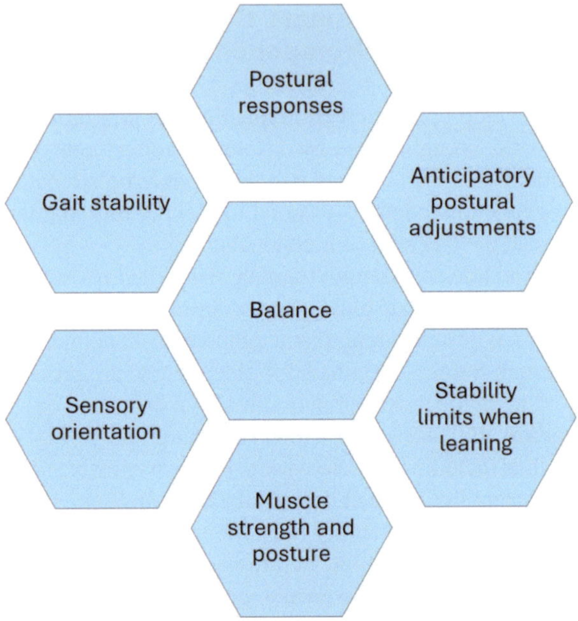

programs when changing base of foot support. Also executive or attentional systems play a role when a person is distracted with multiple visual or auditory cues [10] (Fig. 8.2).

Principles of balance training programs are presented in Table 8.3. Similarly to resistance training principles individualization, progression, and monitoring are keys to improvement.

However, usually solely concentrating on strengthening of muscles is not the most optimal approach to restoring functioning following episodes of ill-health. Instead, combining strength training with other rehabilitative elements targeting balance, mobility skills, nutrition, and pain may be more efficacious in rebuilding the functioning to the level or possibly above the level that the person had prior becoming ill.

Co-impairment is a term parallel to comorbidity and refers to presence of multiple deficits in the functioning of physiological, psychological, or anatomical structure or function. Already several decades ago Duncan et al. suggested that decline in function may be better explained by the accumulation of deficits across multiple functional domains rather than by any single specific impairment [4]. It was found that when the number of impairments (lower and upper extremity, sensory and affective impairments) increased from 0 to 1 to 2 to 3 or more, the proportion of participants experiencing functional dependence doubled from 7% to 14% to 28% to 60%, respectively [37]. In particular, low muscle strength in combination with other physical deficits and related functional limitations may become a critical issue in old age especially when accompanied with acute or chronic health problems. Among older women with disabilities, the odds of severe walking disability were 10

Table 8.3 Principles of balance training [8]

Principle	Description
Individualization	Balance exercises need to be tailored to individual abilities
Progression	The complexity and challenge of balance exercises should progress from static to dynamic tasks
Multidimensional training	Focus on multiple sensory systems (vision, proprioception, vestibular), motor skills, and cognitive functions
Functional relevance	Exercises should mimic daily activities and real-life scenarios
Safety	A safe environment has supports like handrails or spotters. Use of use proper footwear is necessary
Regularity	Balance exercises should be done 2–3 times per week
Strength and flexibility	Strength and flexibility in lower body muscles and joints improves balance
Confidence	Fostering balance confidence stems from achievable goals
Varied techniques	Using balance boards, resistance bands and activities like tai chi, yoga, or dance help promote sustained motivation in balance training
Monitor and adjust	Regularly reassess progress, adjust exercises, and consult healthcare professionals as needed

times greater among those who had both strength and balance impairments compared with those who had only one or the other [26–28]. A potential explanation for this is that people who have impaired function in only one physiological system may be able to compensate for the deficit if they have good capacity in another physiological system.

Studying co-impairments is particularly appropriate in older people because with increasing age, the proportion of those having impairments in multiple physiological systems increases. Co-impairments may arise from the same underlying cause, or they may have different etiologies. For example, we found that among those older people who had visual impairment, their knee extension strength, leg extension power, postural balance, and maximal walking speed were markedly lower than among those who were of same age but did not have visual impairment. It is possible that decreased visual acuity may be a marker of underlying systemic factors or the aging process, which lead to poorer functional capacity, or there may be shared background factors, which lead to decreased vision and lower extremity impairment [13].

It seems reasonable to think that for addressing several co-occurring deficits there needs to be a multicomponent program. Multicomponent training comprises combining of at least three types of training, such as strength, aerobic, balance, coordination, and flexibility training. Recently, a meta-analysis assessing the effectiveness of the programs for improving physical performance including 13 articles with a total of 808 healthy older adults analyzed supported its usefulness for fostering physical performance [14]. Specifically, it was concluded that multicomponent training improves general functional capacity, strength in upper and lower extremities, walking speed, and aerobic capacity. The strength gain in these programs was comparable to gains received in specific strength training interventions. **Multimodal exercise** focuses on balance, endurance, and muscle strength simultaneously by combining two or more types of exercise and sometimes also a nutritional intervention. For older adults with reduced physical capacity, multimodal exercise appears to have a broad effect on improving muscle strength, balance, and physical functioning of the lower extremity and reducing falls. The benefits relative to progressive resistance exercise alone appear wider.

Hospitalizations or injuries among older people often lead to functional decline even though the health condition is cured. Returning to earlier level of functioning may be challenging and require long and progressive rehabilitation programs. One of the early and innovative multicomponent outpatient rehabilitation programs focusing on strength training balance and nutrition among frail, acutely ill older patients was conducted by Dr. Leena Timonen et al. [35]. Their study was designed to improve physical status after hospitalization in terms of muscle strength, gait speed, and balance. Participants were recruited from a geriatric ward of a primary-care health-center hospital. The inclusion criteria were age 75 years or older; female; difficulties in mobility and balance, such as dizziness; or difficulty to walk independently. Training started 1 week after discharge. Training classes were given twice a week, for a 10-week period (20 sessions, 90 min each), and the training sessions were supervised by physiotherapists. Transportation and lunch were provided for each session which typically were carried out in groups including three to eight participants. Each session included a 15-min warm-up, progressive resistance training for knee extension, knee flexion and hip abduction with weight training equipment, lasting about 30 min and with increased resistance. Functional exercises included rising from a chair, hip flexion and extension in a standing position, and rising to a tiptoe position and elbow flexion using light (1–2 kg) ankle or wrist weights. The functional exercises took about 30 min and were followed by a relaxation period of 15 with guided imagery employing the tension-relaxation method. The participants were taught a stretching program to be performed at home later during the same day. This study showed that a multicomponent training program including strength training soon after discharge from a geriatric ward was an effective form of rehabilitation for frail older women with mobility difficulties. The 10-week training program improved maximal voluntary isometric strength, balance, and walking speed in the training group compared to the control group. Some of the improvements were present also at the 3- and 9-month follow-ups. There were two clinically important findings of this study. Maximum walking speed improved, and improvements took place in multiple physiological systems. Walking speed is a powerful predictor of future disability, so improvement in walking speed may indicate a decrease in the risk of disability. Accumulation of impairments in multiple physiological systems creates synergistic disability risk, and consequently alleviating this problem may be especially beneficial for preventing functional decline.

Community-dwelling older persons who survive a hip fracture need special attention to recover appropriate mobility and functional ability, because less than half of them attain their pre-fracture basic mobility and of these less than half regain functioning in more advanced mobility tasks. The complications hindering safe mobility include persistent pain, fear of falling, poor balance, low muscle strength, reduced bone mass, and adverse changes in bone geometry. Thus, older people recovering from a hip fracture are at an increased risk for a recurrent fracture, progressive loss of mobility, disability, and loss of independence.

Some years ago, we conducted a randomized controlled trial to restore functioning of older hip fracture patients [32]. The intervention was designed to be progressive, to be of sufficient duration to allow recovery and regaining mobility, and to follow the principles of overload. Intervention included an individually tailored and home-based mobility training program in addition to standard care. It included five to seven home visits by an experienced physiotherapist; the first three visits took place within 1 month from the hospital discharge and were followed by a visit 3 and 6 months after baseline measurements. There were two partly overlapping phases. Phase I prepared the basis for the physical rehabilitation and physical activity and included evaluation and modification of fall hazards at home, guidance for safe walking including readjustment of walking aids, and information on shoes and anti-slip shoe devices for icy conditions, and written information on assistive devices. In addition, pain assessment and discussions on pain management were incorporated. Phase II included a progressive home exercise program and physical activity counseling. The exercise program comprised strengthening exercises for the lower limbs, balance training in standing position, walking exercises, and stretching. The program was updated to a more challenging one during subsequent five physiotherapist's home visit. Each program took approximately 30 minutes to complete. Strengthening and stretching exercises were done three times a week and balance and walking exercises on 2 to 3 other days in the week. The resistance bands had three different strengths which were individually introduced according to progress.

Approximately 3 months after the baseline, an individual 30-min motivational face-to-face physical activity counseling session was scheduled. The problem-solving method was used to address perceived obstacles to physical activity and to access exercise facilities offered by the municipality. The topics included the level of physical activity before the fracture, the persons' interest in returning to previous activities and beginning to exercise, and the willingness to be active in everyday chores, to exercise on one's own, or to participate in supervised exercise classes. The participant and the physiotherapist together designed a personal physical activity plan, which was supported through three phone contacts and one face-to-face session with 1–2-month interval [32].

The benefits of the intervention compared to standard care were evident. Remarkably, at the end of the 12-month intervention, the participants perceived less difficulties in negotiating stairs compared to the pre-fracture time, a change that differed from the control condition of usual care. Less difficulty in negotiating stairs at 6 and 12 months correlated with better functional balance at 3 and 6 months in the intervention group but not among the control group members. This shows that improvements in the functional building blocks of stair climbing underlie the improvement. To be efficacious in reducing or reversing disability after hip fracture, rehabilitation needs to be individualized, include many components, be progressive, and span a sufficiently long period [31].

The current physical activity guidelines for older Americans provide a list of benefits to functioning and well-being be expected from exercise training including the following: improved sleep, slowed or reduced weight gain, improved bone health, improved physical function, and lower risk of falls and fall-related injuries [20].

The recommended forms of exercise for those who are able:

- At least 150 min–300 min a week of moderate-intensity, or 75 min–150 min a week of vigorous-intensity aerobic physical activity, or an equivalent combination of moderate- and vigorous-intensity aerobic activity. Preferably, aerobic activity should be spread throughout the week.
- Muscle-strengthening activities of moderate or greater intensity that involve all major muscle groups on 2 or more days a week.

When adults with chronic conditions or disabilities are not able to meet the above key guidelines, they should engage in regular physical activity according to their abilities and should avoid inactivity. Adults with chronic conditions or symptoms should be under the care of a health care practitioner. People with chronic conditions can consult a health care professional or physical activity specialist about the types and amounts of activity appropriate for their abilities and chronic conditions.

8.5 Promoting Functional Capacity

Actions fostering functional capacity may be aligned as a framework ranging from policies that help people attain their best possible level of functional capacity to actions that help alleviate disabilities and functional deficits (see Table 8.4). Promoting functional capacity of older people can be categorized into promotional activities, prevention, rehabilitation, and compensation or support services. Additionally, these actions can target the level of organ systems (e.g., muscle strength training), the individual level (e.g., walking exercises), the demands placed on the individual by the environment (e.g., modifying the environment, e.g., with support rails and good lighting), and the level of societal participation (e.g., transportation to a polling station during elections).

Actions targeting individuals aim to improve their capacities to, e.g., see, hear, and walk. As disability stems from a person inability to meet environmental requirements, lowering the environmental demands may also help. Examples of this include home modifications or moving to a less challenging living environment. Challenges in the living environment, such as stairs, may provide a chance to maintain functional capacity if a person manages to negotiate them. Stairs may become an insurmountable barrier if the individual's capacity is insufficient to mount the steps. Societal participation can be enhanced by seeking solutions that enable individuals to participate in activities according to their goals regardless of their functional capacity. Examples include transportation services or volunteer assistance to polling stations or civil society meetings.

Table 8.4 Different levels for promoting functional capacity of older people

Category	Explanation
Promotion	Actions that increase activity, participation, and well-being, thereby growing the functional capacity reserve. Examples include the activities of sports and pensioner organizations, the cultural sector, social capital, health-promoting lifestyles, and the early and effective treatment of diseases. Legislation or insurance guaranteeing access to certain services, like timely access to care or the policies increasing physical activity for all, also falls into this category
Prevention	Actions to reduce or eliminate risks that might increase the chances of progression to disability. Information dissemination to the general population or specific healthcare measures targeted at particular groups. Preventive home visits and screenings are examples
Rehabilitation	A systematic process for maintaining and improving functional capacity and work ability with the help of professionals A set of interventions needed when a person is experiencing or is likely to develop limitations in everyday functioning For example: physiotherapy, occupational therapy or speech therapy
Compensation	Strategies to offset declines in functional capacity by doing things differently, using assistive devices, or modifying the living environment. Examples include eyeglasses, hearing aids, walkers, and other technological solutions that improve safety. Social and health services play a role by providing support for activities individuals can no longer perform independently, helping to reduce the demands of the environment

8.6 Promotional Actions for Physical Functioning

Promotional activities to increase activity, participation, and well-being can be thought of as increasing the "functional capacity reserve." Activities by sports organizations and pensioner organizations and the cultural sector can be seen as promotional. Social capital, health-promoting lifestyles, an active lifestyle, and physical activity, as well as good and early treatment of diseases, fall into this category. The course of earlier life, such as education, work, and social relationships, can outreach the present and underlie good functional capacity in old age. Legislation can also be seen as part of this category. For example, laws can guarantee the availability of certain services, such as timely access to care. When there is sufficient research evidence on the harmfulness of a health habit, it can even be prohibited by law. Examples of such laws include the ban on smoking in workplaces and in public places that came into effect in the 1990s. Unquestionably protective behaviors may also be obliged by law. An example of this concerns the mandatory use of seat belts in a car, which has been in effect since 1970s. In general, prohibitive laws are problematic in terms of enforcement and individual freedom. Laws related to smoking and seat belts have been more readily accepted than, for example, the prohibition of alcohol.

Also, environmental facilitators for health-enhancing behaviors influence older people's functioning. We identified environmental facilitators for outdoor walking and examined their association with the development of walking difficulty in community-dwelling older people using a prospective study design with a 3.5-year follow-up time among 261 community-dwelling people aged 75–81 years. Participants were able to walk 0.5 km without difficulty at the baseline. Environmental facilitators for outdoor walking were features in one's home which make it easy to access the outdoors, having a park or other green area within a walking distance from home, having outdoor recreational facilities within a walking distance from home, having features attracting to outdoor activities in one's nearby environment, and perceiving the surrounding environment or facilities nearby as motivating factors for physical activity. Self-reported difficulty in walking 0.5 km was assessed every 6 months. Of the participants, 46% developed walking difficulty during the follow-up. Having a park or other green area within a walking distance from home was the most frequently reported facilitator. Environmental facilitators decreased the risk for developing walking difficulty. The hazard ratio per item was 0.86, (95% confidence interval 0.73–1.02). The results indicate that the mobility of older community-dwelling people may be promoted with outdoor recreational facilities that are easy to access and located within a walking distance from home [5].

Attending to the walkability of neighborhoods may be a feasible way to promote older people's possibilities to participate in different activities. Neighborhood walkability describes the environment's suitability for walking to different destinations. Walkability is often operationalized based on land use, population density, and street connectivity, which may be combined to form a walkability index, with a higher value indicating better walkability. Walkable environments support older people's independence and mobility, give them an opportunity to maintain social networks, and promote their community participation. Factors such as high population density land use diversity and proximity to destinations may enable community participation and mobility outside the home for older people. In addition, higher walkability has been found to be associated with higher physical activity among older adults [21]. In our study among 848 community living people aged 75–90 years, we found that living in the highest walkability area, such as the city center, was associated with frequent participation in cultural or other individual activities but with lower participation in outdoor recreation. Participants with intact walking or using walking modifications were more likely than those with walking difficulties to participate frequently in leisure activities. In the 4-year follow-up, living in a middle or the highest compared to the lowest walkability area predicted higher participation in cultural or other individual activities [38].

8.7 Prevention of Functional Decline

The prevention of functional decline may in practice overlap with rehabilitation, especially when the intervention concerns people who have ill-health. Prevention of functional limitations can, however, target the entire population through information dissemination, physical activity classes, or specific groups through different organizations or healthcare measures.

Physical activity provides a sustainable means for preventing mobility limitation and further disability among older people with chronic conditions. However, research-based evidence on cost-effective strategies and context where best to increase physical activity participation in old age is still scarce. Exercise promotion strategies have used verbal advice, written prescription, telephone support, or mailed booklets, but the long-term effects of these programs on behavior change and disability outcomes are less studied and not entirely convincing. Many older people have regular contact with healthcare providers and healthcare organizations which could serve as a resource for physical activity promotion among older people. Ideally, physical activity advice should be individually tailored based on illnesses, functional limitations, personal preferences, and potential to exercise. Features of the physical and social environment and opportunities provided for older individuals to exercise should be considered. An effective physical activity counseling approach needs to comprise practical solutions and support systems for adherence.

The general idea of preventive actions is that for the most cost-effective results, an intervention should be targeted at people who will most likely receive benefits from it, i.e., those who do not yet have the functional limitation but are at risk of developing it. For physical activity counseling, people with a low level of physical activity and first signs of mobility limitation may form a fruitful target group. Almost 20 years ago, we conducted one of the first studies on physical activity counselling with multilevel outcomes: behavior change, physiological impairments, functional limitations, and disability. Physical activity counseling is an educational intervention. We considered that cognitively intact older people who were able to move outdoors independently but were physically sedentary would be the group that would most likely benefit from physical activity counseling. Consequently, the inclusion criteria were set as follows: (a) the ability to walk at least 0.5 km without assistance, (b) only moderately physically active or sedentary, (c) no memory impairment, (d) no medical contraindications for physical activity, and (e) informed consent to participate [15].

The intervention consisted of an individualized face-to-face meeting followed by telephone contacts every 4 months for 2 years, with the aim to increase participation in specific physical activities and habitual physical activity. The counseling approach went along the strategies developed based on social cognitive theory of health behavior change. The counseling technique was motivational and promoted self-efficacy for more active physical behavior. The participants were motivated to change by helping them notice the discrepancy between the present and the desired level of physical activity. The counselor facilitated problem-solving tactics to tackle the barriers to change and foster a plan for more active physical behavior. For those interested in joining a supervised exercise, referrals were given to inexpensive exercise classes for older people available in our community. Participants were also encouraged to exercise on their own. After the face-to-face counseling session, the counselor supported the compliance and behavior change through regular phone contacts over the 2-year intervention.

After 2 years, the prevalence of physical activities in the intervention group vs. control group was as follows: supervised calisthenics training 20 vs. 16%, walking for fitness 69 vs. 62%, weight training 13 vs. 8%, and water aerobics 19 vs. 7%. One and half years after the intervention ended, the intervention effect was still evident. The subgroup analyses suggested that physical activity counseling may be most efficacious among people with intact mobility, while those having early manifest mobility limitations may not benefit from it [30]. For mobility, the outcome measures were the perceived difficulty in advanced (walking 2 km) and basic (walking 0.5 km) mobility. Data were gathered semiannually during the intervention and the 1.5-year postintervention follow-up. In the intervention group, the proportion of participants with difficulties in advanced mobility at the beginning and end of the intervention was 34% and 38%, respectively. In the control group, the corresponding proportions were 32% and 45%. The treatment effect was significant at the 2-year follow-up (odds ratio 0.84, 95% confidence interval 0.70–0.99; $P = 0.04$) and remained significant 1.5 years postintervention (0.82, 0.68–0.99; $P = 0.04$). The effect on basic mobility postintervention was parallel but nonsignificant (0.87, 0.69–1.09; $P = 0.22$; [17]). Majority of the beneficial effect of the intervention on mobility took place via the prevention of new difficulty among those without difficulty at baseline, whereas the ameliorating effect on those with baseline difficulty was smaller. The physical activity counseling intervention had no effect on IADL disability, although it prevented incident IADL disability [41]. Older people who have symptoms of mobility limitations may require more support and a more structured and intensive intervention for better compliance and recovery.

Our results suggest that to benefit from interventions aiming to prevent functional limitation, the participants need to have enough resources to independently follow the course of the program, i.e., they need cognitive and physical capacities and an environment that supports the program. A recent meta-analysis established that physical activity counselling and exercise referral interventions in primary care are in general effective and can be delivered by healthcare providers working with the primary provider and that many different behavior change strategies may be used to promote physical activity [19].

More research is needed on which groups benefit most from the prevention of functional limitations and which measures are most effective. Often the risk of functional decline coincides with hospitalization, particularly among older people. In a large study among people aged 70 years and older hospitalizations were documented for 72% of those developing catastrophic disability and for 48% of those developing progressive disability during the year when the disability was detected. In the corresponding year, only 15% of those who were stable with no disability and 22% of those with some disabilities were hospitalized [6]. Catastrophic disability refers to a trajectory where functional decline happens fast, while progressive disability refers to a gradual development over a longer period. These results suggest that interventions aimed at reducing the functional consequences of diseases could have a large impact on reduction of severe disability if appropriately timed and planned. Even an acute, curable illness requiring a few days of hospitalization can propel a decline in functioning, especially among those whose reserve capacity of functioning has already reached an at-risk level. Approximately 30% of hospitalized older adults experience hospital-associated functional decline. Exercise interventions that promote in-hospital activity may prevent deconditioning and thereby maintain physical function during hospitalization. Consequently, appropriate evaluation, counseling, and rehabilitation during and after hospitalization could be a feasible way to promote recuperation of functional capacity.

Hospital discharge is a complex, sometimes rushed, process often driven by the pressure to reduce hospital stays. A recent meta-analysis of the effects of exercise interventions categorized into rehabilitation-related activities (interventions designed to increase physical activity or functional recovery but not following a specified exercise protocol); structured exercise (interventions that included an exercise intervention protocol but did not include progressive resistance training); and progressive resistance exercise (interventions that included an element of progressive resistance training). The authors concluded that exercise may have no clinically important effect on independence in activities of daily living at discharge from hospital compared to controls. The effects of exercise on functional mobility at discharge from the hospital compared to controls were modest and provided very low-certainty evidence [9].

Discharge from hospital may be complicated by overwhelming information to the person being discharged. Recently, a Delphi study identified 41 factors that are critical to ensure the mobility of older adults transitioning from hospital to home in the community [12]. These factors were categorized into cognitive (e.g., executive function, visuospatial function), environmental (e.g., public transport, support systems), personal (e.g., age, history of readmissions), physical (e.g., muscle strength, balance, vision), psychological (e.g., motivation, fear of falls), and social (e.g., loneliness, living situation) determinants. It is probably unfeasible to assess all these factors in hospitals; however, this outline may serve as a basis for future less extensive screening instrument for safe discharge.

It is important to develop counseling and rehabilitation related to discharge for elderly individuals. Common symptoms and ailments in old age, such as urinary incontinence, depressive symptoms, falls, fatigue, anemia, or pain, increase the risk of functional decline. Targeted correct measures can slow down the decline in functional capacity. To prevent functional limitations, it is essential to address risk factors and maintain functional capacity through counseling and rehabilitation. Screening for risks related to functional capacity or functional capacity assessments have been tried, but evidence of their effectiveness is limited. The problem also lies in the diversity of assessment and screening methods, indicating a need for development in this field. The development and standardization of functional capacity assessment methods and subsequent interventions following observed deficiencies are prerequisites for the effectiveness of prevention and rehabilitation of disabilities. Home visits or phone screening could offer an opportunity to early detection of individuals at increased risk of functional decline, who would benefit from preventive measures. However, prevention targeting only risk groups is likely not sufficient; promoting functional capacity upstream is a matter for the entire population.

8.8 Rehabilitation

Rehabilitation is a systematic process in which the rehabilitees maintain and improve their functional capacity and work ability with the help of professionals. Physical rehabilitation refers to interventions exercising the body. Geriatric rehabilitation has recently gained a lot of scientific attention. Older residents of long-term care form the frailest section of the population, having substantial healthcare and social care needs. In developed countries, long-term care for older people is often provided in institutional settings for those with physical or mental conditions that exclude independent living. There is considerable research evidence on the effectiveness of regaining functioning in different organ systems, such as muscle strength, balance, and mobility. Muscle strength and balance can be improved even in old age, but the effects are small. However, the evidence is less clear for functional limitations and disability. In all, interventions in long-term care provide preliminary evidence that physical rehabilitation interventions may be associated with significant improvements across various measures of physical and mental functioning, without increasing the mortality risk in old care-home residents [3]. However, most studies have been conducted in ideal circumstances. They require replication in routine care and everyday practice to determine external validity and direct comparison between different interventions. At present, there is no clear indication of the optimum type of intervention, but some interesting models have been published.

One of the first studies to test multimodal physical rehabilitation after an acute hospitalization was a 10-week training program after hospitalization designed to improve lower limb muscle strength, gait speed, and balance. The training started 1 week after discharge. Ninety-minute training group classes were given twice a week, for a 10-week period in the health center gym, where participants were provided with transportation and lunch was served after each training session. The training was progressive strength training and included functional exercises for balance and mobility. Control group received usual care. The 10-week training program improved maximal voluntary isometric strength, balance, and walking speed in the training group compared to the control group. Some of the improvements were present also at the 3- and 9-month follow-ups [35]. However, this rather short intervention did not significantly improve independence in ADL or IADL [35]. There were no differences between the intervention and control groups in the mean individual healthcare costs, in the social welfare costs, or in the fall-related healthcare costs [36]. This study showed that exercise classes including strength training and functional exercises soon after discharge from a geriatric ward were an effective and feasible form of rehabilitation for impairments and functional limitations as discussed earlier, but among frail older women with mobility difficulties ADL and IADL did not change. It is worth noting, that such a program did not increase health care costs.

For older adults with reduced physical capacity, multimodal exercise is effective in improving muscle strength of the lower extremity, dynamic standing balance, gait speed, and chair stand. In addition, multimodal exercise is effective in reducing falls but does not improve activities of daily living. Multimodal exercise appears to have a broad effect on improving muscle strength, balance, and physical functioning of the lower extremity and reducing falls relative to progressive resistance exercise alone [16].

8.9 Compensation

Compensation refers to a situation where people acquire and start using new or previously unused resources which help them continue doing meaningful activities in the face of functional loss. In this context, compensation means that a person can offset declines in functional capacity by doing things differently, using aids, or modifying or changing the living environment. For example, glasses, hearing aids, and walkers are commonly used to improve mobility safety, social interaction, and participation opportunities. The development and testing of technological solutions are active research areas, especially the development of customer-oriented technological solutions. Social and health services support the home living of individuals with reduced functional capacity by aiding with activities they can no longer perform independently. In addition, modifying the home environment to reduce physical mobility barriers and promote safety will facilitate independent and safe life at the home. Typically, the first step needs to include assistance with hygiene, medication, and transport. Problems in transport are among the most common challenges experienced by older people with functional limitations and disabilities.

Some years ago, we conducted a study where volunteers were recruited to assist older people with mobility limitations in out-of-home mobility. First, we conducted a narrative review to examine the association of formal voluntary work and personal well-being among older people doing the voluntary work and those being served. Studies mainly used data from large datasets with only limited information about volunteering, which limited more detailed analyses. We concluded that randomized controlled trials were needed to study the effect of voluntary work on those being served because no studies were identified that had examined whether it was possible to quantify the well-being benefits for those people who were served [40].

Volunteering We realized that the current healthcare policy favoring home care rather than institutional care had led to a situation where increasingly frail people who are not able to access the outdoors independently continue living in their own homes. Providing opportunities for participation also for older people with difficulty accessing the outdoors independently is important and could promote their well-being. Volunteers could facilitate out-of-home activity for people who have difficulty accessing the outdoors independently. We also realized that people, who have recently retired, are looking for ways to be active and engage with their communities. They could be interested in volunteering, given that the activity is attractive to them and well organized and that volunteers are trained and supported.

Our goal was to examine whether an out-of-home activity intervention delivered by older volunteers improves quality of life of older people in home care who perceive difficulty entering the outdoors independently. Our intervention idea was based on co-production of well-being among older people, in terms that the volunteer and the person served would together increase the well-being of each other when both possess productive roles. Volunteers assisted older adults with severe mobility limitations to various out-of-home activities based on their interests and needs. Each of the volunteers was individually introduced by the study coordinator to a participant. The selection of these pairs was discretionary and based, e.g., on the closeness of their homes. The volunteer, the participant, and the coordinator discussed together about the out-of-home activity interests of the participant and made an activity plan for the intervention period. The interventions included activities such as going to walks and visiting places of interest (e.g., the harbor, parks, art and craft exhibitions, the cemetery) or cultural events or taking care of daily errands. The volunteer and the participant met once a week for a 3-month period. During the intervention, volunteers met once a month to discuss their experiences. After the waiting list control period, the control group members were offered a similar intervention. The intervention improved the physical capacity subscore of the quality-of-life scale. In addition, the mood state of those with minor depressive symptoms improved [22]. The results suggest that volunteers may contribute to promoting the quality-of life of old people with severe mobility limitations living in the community [29].

Subsequently the benefits of volunteering on the health of those served have gained more interest. A recent systematic review and meta-analysis identified 28 studies that evaluated the effects of unpaid volunteer interventions on health-related outcomes among older people. The study supports the role of volunteers to increase physical activity levels and to improve older people's subjective ratings of physical health, without harm. The findings aligned with the WHO call to action on aging. Policymakers, clinical leaders, health system planners, volunteer organizations, and others should consider the role of volunteers in health system planning for aging populations to add relational support, improve connection with social and healthcare systems, and augment health professional resources and services [18].

To ensure a positive volunteering experience for those helping and those receiving help, the responsible organizations need to establish a quality system for the volunteer work in terms of supervising and supporting the volunteers. Typically, features of good quality in volunteering follow principles of customer-friendliness, confidentiality, ethics, and mentoring/supervising the volunteers. Customer-friendliness emphasizes satisfying the needs of both the volunteers and those being served. Confidentiality refers to protecting personal information and not sharing details of health, place of residence, lifestyle, or family with anybody outside the team. Ethics in volunteering typically relate to promoting positive elements, such as humanity and equality. The goal of mentoring is to strengthen the volunteer's identity and development in their tasks. Central aspects of mentoring the volunteers working with older people include sharing experiences and feelings with peers. Most volunteers strive to help others, obtain new interesting experiences, and thus create mutual benefits with the person served. It is worth noting that in addition to providing training and supporting the performance of volunteer work, also dignified completion of volunteering needs to be made possible (see Table 8.5 for summary).

New Operational Models Promoting the functional capacity of older people requires the implementation of new operational models and research aimed at changing existing practices (Table 8.6). The speed of knowledge transfer has been found to be influenced by (1) how the innovation is perceived, (2) the characteristics of the individuals who accept or reject the innovation, and (3) environmental factors such as leadership, governance, incentives, and communication. The benefits brought by new knowledge significantly impact the adoption and implementation into practice. If new information leads to unpleasant or laborious changes, very strong evidence is needed to alter practices. Furthermore, the information must be compatible with values, beliefs, history, and the current needs of individuals. Moreover, the simplicity of the information affects its perception. Simpler innovations spread more easily than complex ones. A good example of this is the spread of strength training as a form of physical exercise and rehabilitation among older people and their service systems. In Finland, the national "Strength for Old Age" program, has made strength training accessible to everyone. The program is based on clear research evidence of the benefits of strength training for functional capacity and the minimal adverse effects, with clearly identifiable results and an easily understandable intervention. The goal of the "Strength for Old Age" program is to

Table 8.5 Summary of essential aspects of high-quality volunteering

Aspect	Description
Quality system	Organizations should establish systems to supervise and support volunteers
Customer-friendliness	Focusing on meeting the needs of both volunteers and those being served
Confidentiality	Ensuring personal information is protected and not shared outside the team
Ethics	Promoting humanity, equality, and other positive values
Mentoring/ supervising	Strengthen volunteers' identity and development through peer experience and emotional support
Training and support	Provide proper training and ongoing support for volunteer tasks
Completion of volunteering	Ensure a dignified end to the volunteering experience

Table 8.6 Components for evaluating the success of implementing a new operational model

Component
Was the target population reached?
How many stakeholders adopted the new operational model?
How successful is the use of the new operational model?
How permanent was the change at the individual and population levels?

increase leg muscle strength and improve balance among older individuals, thereby preventing mobility restrictions and maintaining independence. The program is founded on the government's policy decision on the development of health-promoting physical activity. The long-term goal of the program was to disseminate and produce information, gain experiences, and create operational practices that become a permanent part of the daily lives and well-being services of older people. An important part of the "Strength for Old Age" program is the local projects implemented by various organizations, where exercise programs based on researched knowledge are carried out in ways that are well-suited to each area. The program also encourages new forms of collaboration as a criterion for financial support.

An aging society and service system require researched knowledge and continuing education based on researched knowledge to develop their operations. There are no ready-made solutions for the systematic utilization of knowledge. It is known that practices can only be changed through measures involving employees, management, and the entire organization. In promoting the functional capacity of older people, the civil society could be crucial in utilizing knowledge from basic research and highlighting development needs arising from social practices.

References

1. Bhasin S, Travison TG, Manini TM, et al. Sarcopenia definition: the position statements of the sarcopenia definition and outcomes consortium. J Am Geriatr Soc. 2020;68:1410–8.
2. Clark BC, Manini TM. Sarcopenia ≠ Dynapenia. J Gerontol Med Sci. 2008;63:829–34.
3. Crocker T, Forster A, Young J, et al. Physical rehabilitation for older people in long-term care. Cochrane Database Syst Rev. 2013;2:CD004294.
4. Duncan PW, Chandler J, Studensky S, et al. How do physiological components of balance affect mobility in elderly men? Arch Phys Med Rehabil. 1993;74:1343–9.
5. Eronen J, von Bonsdorff M, Rantakokko M, Rantanen T. Environmental facilitators for outdoor walking and development of walking difficulty in community-dwelling older adults. Eur J Ageing. 2013;11:67–75.
6. Ferrucci L, Guralnik JM, Pahor M, et al. Hospital diagnoses, medicare charges, and nursing home admissions in the year when older persons become severely disabled. JAMA. 1997;277:728–34.
7. Fiatarone MA, Marks EC, Ryan ND, Meredith CN, Lipsitz LA, Evans WJ. High-intensity strength training in nonagenarians. Effects on skeletal muscle. JAMA. 1990;13(263):3029–34.
8. Halvarsson A, Dohrn IM, Ståhle A. Taking balance training for older adults one step further: the rationale for and a description of a proven balance training program. Clin Rehabil. 2015;29:417–25.
9. Hartley P, Keating JL, Jeffs KJ, et al. Exercise for acutely hospitalized older medical patients. Cochrane Database Syst Rev. 2022;11:CD005955.
10. Horak FB, Wrisley DM, Frank J. The balance evaluation systems test (BESTest) to differentiate balance deficits. Phys Ther. 2009;89:484–98.
11. Kallman DA, Plato CC, Tobin JD. The role of muscle strength loss in the age-related decline in grip strength: cross-sectional and longitudinal perspectives. J Gerontol. 1990;45A:M82–8.
12. Kalu ME, Dal Bello-Haas V, Griffin M, et al. What mobility factors are critical to include in a comprehensive mobility discharge assessment framework for older adults transitioning from hospital-to-home in the community? An international e-Delphi study. Disabil Rehabil. 2023;46:2808–20.

13. Kulmala J, Sipilä S, Tiainen K, Pärssinen O, Koskenvuo M, Kaprio J, Rantanen T. Vision in relation to lower extremity deficit in older women: cross-sectional and longitudinal study. Aging Clin Exp Res. 2012;24:461–7.
14. Labata-Lezaun N, González-Rueda V, Llurda-Almuzara L, et al. Effectiveness of multicomponent training on physical performance in older adults: a systematic review and meta-analysis. Arch Gerontol Geriatr. 2023;104:104838.
15. Leinonen R, Heikkinen E, Hirvensalo M, et al. Customer-oriented counseling for physical activity in older people: study protocol and selected baseline results of a randomized-controlled trial (ISRCTN 07330512). Scand J Med Sci Sports. 2007;17:156–64.
16. Liu C, Chang WP, de Carvalho A, et al. Effects of physical exercise in older adults with reduced physical capacity: meta-analysis of resistance exercise and multimodal exercise. Int J Rehabn Res. 2017;40:303–14.
17. Mänty M, Heinonen A, Leinonen R, et al. Long-term effect of physical activity counseling on mobility limitation among older people: a randomized controlled study. J Gerontol Biol Sci Med Sci A. 2009;64:83–9.
18. Moore A, Motagh S, Sadeghirad B, et al. Volunteer impact on health-related outcomes for seniors: a systematic review and meta-analysis. Can Geriatr J. 2021;24:44–72.
19. Otmanowski JA, Chase JD. Systematic review and meta-analysis of primary care-based physical activity interventions among older adults. J Aging Phys Act. 2022;30:842–56.
20. Piercy KL, Troiano RP, Ballard RM, et al. The physical activity guidelines for Americans. JAMA. 2018;320:2020–8.
21. Portegijs E, Keskinen KE, Tsai LT, et al. Physical limitations, walkability, perceived environmental facilitators and physical activity of older adults in Finland. Int J Environ Res Public Health. 2017;14:333.
22. Rantakokko M, Pakkala I, Äyräväinen I, Rantanen T. The effect of out-of-home activity intervention delivered by volunteers on depressive symptoms among older people with severe mobility limitations: a randomized controlled trial. Aging Ment Health. 2015;19:231–8.
23. Rantanen T, Guralnik JM. Ferrucci L et al Coimpairments as predictors of severe walking disability in older women. J Am Geriatr Soc. 2001;49:21–7.
24. Rantanen T, Guralnik JM, Izmirlian G, et al. Association of muscle strength with maximum walking speed in disabled older women. Am J Phys Med Rehabil. 1998a;77:299–305.
25. Rantanen T, Masaki K, Foley D, Izmirlian G, White L, Guralnik JM. Grip strength changes over 27 yr in Japanese American men. J Appl Physiol. 1998b;85:2047–53.
26. Rantanen T, Guralnik JM, Ferrucci L, et al. Coimpairments: strength and balance as predictors of severe walking disability. J Gerontol Med Sci. 1999a;54A:M172–6.
27. Rantanen T, Guralnik JM, Foley D, et al. Midlife hand grip strength as a predictor of old age disability. JAMA. 1999b;281:558–60.
28. Rantanen T, Guralnik JM, Sakari-Rantala R, et al. Disability, physical activity, and muscle strength in older women: the women's health and aging study. Arch Phys Med Rehabil. 1999c;80:130–5.
29. Rantanen T, Äyräväinen I, Eronen J, et al. The effect of an outdoor activities' intervention delivered by older volunteers on the quality of life of older people with severe mobility limitations: a randomized controlled trial. Aging Clin Exp Res. 2015;27:161–9.
30. Rasinaho M, Hirvensalo M, Törmäkangas T, et al. Effect of physical activity counseling on physical activity of older people in Finland (ISRCTN 07330512). Health Promot Int. 2012;27:463–74.
31. Salpakoski A, Törmäkangas T, Edgren J, et al. Effects of a multicomponent home-based physical rehabilitation program on mobility recovery after hip fracture: a randomized controlled trial. J Am Med Dir Assoc. 2014;15:361–8.
32. Sipilä S, Salpakoski A, Edgren J, et al. Promoting mobility after hip fracture (ProMo): study protocol and selected baseline results of a year-long randomized controlled trial among community-dwelling older people. BMC Musculoskelet Disord. 2011;12:277.

33. Soysal P, Hurst C, Demurtas J, et al. Handgrip strength and health outcomes: umbrella review of systematic reviews with meta-analyses of observational studies. J Sport Health Sci. 2021;10:290–5.
34. Stenholm S, Alley D, Bandinelli S, et al. The effect of obesity combined with low muscle strength on decline in mobility in older persons: results from the InCHIANTI study. Int J Obes. 2009;33:635–44.
35. Timonen L, Rantanen T, Mäkinen E, et al. Effects of a group-based exercise program on functional abilities in frail older women after hospital discharge. Aging Clin Exp Res. 2006;18:50–6.
36. Timonen L, Rantanen T, Mäkinen E, et al. Cost analysis of an exercise program for older women with respect to social welfare and healthcare costs: a pilot study. Scand J Med Sci Sports. 2008;18:783–9.
37. Tinetti ME, Inouye SK, Gill TM, et al. Shared risk factors for falls, incontinence, and functional dependence. JAMA. 1995;273:1348–53.
38. Tuomola EM, Keskinen KE, Viljanen A, et al. Neighborhood walkability, walking difficulties, and participation in leisure activities among older people: a cross-sectional study and 4-year follow-up of a subsample. J Aging Health. 2024;36:367–78.
39. Viljanen A, Kulmala J, Rantakokko M, et al. Fear of falling and coexisting sensory difficulties as predictors of mobility decline in older women. J Gerontol A Biol Sci Med Sci. 2012;67:1230–7.
40. von Bonsdorff MB, Rantanen T. Benefits of formal voluntary work among older people. A review. Aging Clin Exp Res. 2011;23:162–9.
41. von Bonsdorff MB, Leinonen R, Kujala UM, et al. Effect of physical activity counseling on disability in older people: a 2-year randomized controlled trial. J Am Geriatr Soc. 2008;56:2188–94.

9 Life Course Influences on Growing Old and Healthy Aging

Abstract

When people enter old age, they have already lived a long life. Some people started their life in an auspicious situation, while for others the beginning of life may have happened in less favorable circumstances. The early life situations may steer people to different educational and occupational trajectories; however, these developments are not necessarily inevitable. People make decisions and dedicate themselves to reaching their goals. The historical, social, economic, and natural context offers opportunities while also presenting barriers for realizing one's ambitions. Factoring in individual strengths and weaknesses together with the physical and social circumstances enriches the multidimensionality of research on life course influences growing old. Sorting out the relative importance of various influences is a challenge. Life course approach is useful for understanding the wide variation in aging patterns between individuals. This chapter will discuss different approaches to the life course studies on growing old.

Life course research is based on a set of five basic principles defined by Elder et al. [9]. First, human development and aging are not restricted to specific life stages but continue throughout life span. Second, people have agency, which refers to taking actions and making choices that influence their lives within the limits of environmental, social, and historical contexts. Third, individual lives are embedded in and affected by historical time and place. Fourth, the identical events and actions can have different consequences conditional on the age when they take place. Fifth, people do not live alone but influence each other through mutually dependent relationships.

The life course approach to functional capacity in old age suggests that the pattern of change in functioning depends on (1) the peak function attained earlier in life

T. Rantanen, *Advancing Research on Active Aging and Participation*, https://doi.org/10.1007/978-3-031-94702-5_9

due to developmental processes, (2) earlier influences, and (3) contemporary influences. The old age phenotypes result from intrinsic and extrinsic exposures across the life course and the corresponding responses. Life course studies of growing old involve examining the lived life through biological, psychological, social, economic, and historical factors. This interdisciplinary approach helps to understand how different life experiences and transitions influence growing old. Not all individuals begin their life with equal assets. A healthy start and ideal childhood development build up health reserve and contribute to attaining higher intrinsic capacity for functioning. As years go by, retaining good functioning and building a propitious life is more probable among people who experienced optimal developmental patterns that led to higher maximum capacities compared to people with less than ideal early development. In real life, a wide set of social factors influence the framework of development and aging. The life course approach emphasizes that the health and functioning at a specific age is not isolated but is a product of what happened earlier and a sign of what may happen later [33]. For an outline of external and internal influences working across life span, see Fig. 9.1.

In the integrated model, six phases of life are outlined: conception, pre-natal, pre-pubertal, pubertal, maturity, and senescence. The model also presents external and internal environments, which interact with each other. The interactions may operate through direct physiological changes, for example, weight loss happens due to reduced food intake—either intentional or unintentional. These dynamic systems can operate in negative and positive ways. They may maintain body homeostasis or increase instability. Aging does not happen in a uniform way in all systems, but rather has stochastic features. For some, age changes may be more dominant in one system, e.g., cognitive functioning, while for others, physical decline may be more prominent [3].

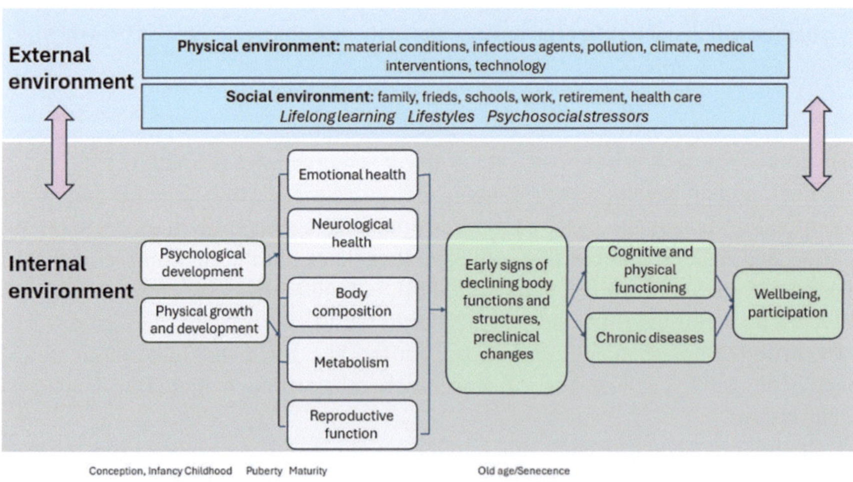

Fig. 9.1 An integrated life course model of aging. (This figure is simplified from an original figure by [18])

9.1 Life Course Epidemiology of Healthy Aging

The idea of healthy aging comes true when we can observe survival to old age, delay in the onset of age-dependent diseases, and optimum functioning for the maximum period. The promotion of healthy aging requires policies and actions concerning all age groups. Research on predictors of healthy aging require longitudinal data. Life course epidemiology studies healthy aging in the context of social, behavioral, and biological pathways between earlier experiences and exposures and healthy aging phenotypes. Exposures to risk factors during gestation, infancy, childhood, adolescence, or young adulthood may lead to physiological or psychological adaptations that are protective in the short term but form long-term biological chains of risk that accelerate aging or increase the risk of disorders in later life. Social chains of risk or protective chains operate throughout life partly via educational and other learning experiences and lead to adult socioeconomic circumstances that affect aging and disease risk through exposures to causal factors in later life. Each life stage includes physical hazards, behaviors with known or suspected biological pathways, and stressful life conditions that affect biological resources through currently only partially understood psychosocial processes [4]. A graph describing the different analytical models of life course epidemiology is shown in Fig. 9.2.

The *sensitive period model* posits that during some periods across the life course, an exposure has a stronger effect, either negative or positive, on health and aging than if it took place during other periods. Examples of such sensitive periods include gestation, infancy, and life transitions. For instance, a lead exposure during early childhood, a critical period for brain development, can result in permanent cognitive impairments that persist into adulthood. Identifying potential sensitive and critical periods for disease risk factors across the life course aids in the optimal timing of preventive interventions. On the other hand, certain aspects of the brain structure

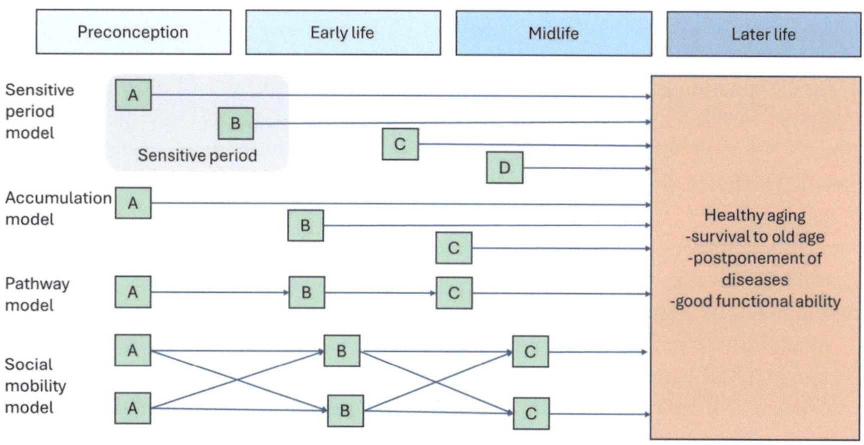

Fig. 9.2 Theoretical life-course models for healthy aging. A, C, and D are exposures at different times during life span. Arrows indicate effects. (Modified from [17, 33])

and function that develop during favorable sensitive periods can buffer against the cognitive decline by contributing to building up cognitive reserve [31]. Education is, for example, one of the most powerful cognitive interventions reaching practically all.

So far, only a few studies have investigated the association between infant motor development, a process that signifies a sensitive period for neurological development and adult cognitive functioning. One of the few reports comes from the 1946 British Birth Cohort study, which found that the earlier the infants learned to stand, the better was their executive functioning in adulthood [26]. Executive functioning comprises processes and skills relating to selecting and pursuing goals. This involves problem-solving, planning, and dealing with emotions—operations that can remarkably contribute to quality of life or even health. Some other studies have reported findings in line with that study, but the follow-ups rarely reach into older ages. Studying prospectively the relationship between infant development and motor milestones as predictors of older age cognitive and physical functioning requires very long follow-ups, but such studies would most likely further the understanding of early potentially modifiable predictors of healthy aging.

One of the few studies with data extending from birth to old age is called the Helsinki Birth Cohort study, which comprises 8760 persons who were born during 1934–1944 in Helsinki and who as infants had attended child welfare clinics and resided in Finland in 1971. Of these people, a subsample was randomly selected to take part in a cognitive ability test when they were on average 64 years old. Subsequently, a subgroup of 398 individual were identified who had valid data in their charts on age when they learned to walk. The children had visited the welfare clinics with their mothers on average 11 times between birth and 2 years of age. The age when the child learned to walk without support was asked from the mothers during their visits to the clinics and was registered in months. The subgroup with data on age first walking did not differ in terms of birth weight from those who had no records of age first walked. In the age- and gender-adjusted models of test results at age 64 years, later attainment of learning to walk lengthened the reaction times in all cognitive performance tasks tested as expressed per each month's delay: 11.0% in simple reaction time task, 14.8% in choice reaction task, and 14.8% for working memory. Further adjustment for father's occupational status and own highest attained education and for adult occupational status did not attenuate the associations [27]. Hence, the effects of earlier attainment of motor skills seem to track over to better cognitive functioning in early old age. This study suggested that timing of motor development in infancy, which has been identified as a period of rapid brain growth, may track over to cognitive performance in early old age possibly due to development of cognitive reserve.

In addition to cognitive development, the early development of musculoskeletal system and body composition may also track into healthy aging. Maintaining musculoskeletal function for the maximal period and preventing musculoskeletal disorders are important aspects of healthy aging. There is evidence that an adverse intrauterine environment can affect muscle histology in animals. In humans, one evident manifestation of less-than-optimal prenatal development is low birth weight.

Several studies have reported that low birth weight correlates with lower muscle strength later in life [8]. Fetal programming, also known as developmental programming or the Barker hypothesis, pertains to the fetal origins of adult diseases. This hypothesis is based on epidemiological data that show that low birth weight due to maternal malnutrition has long-term effects on adult health. Fetal nutrient deficiency can result from maternal malnutrition, reduced placenta efficiency, adolescence pregnancy, and closely spaced pregnancy. Compared to brain and heart, skeletal muscle and fat have a lower priority for nutrition repartitioning, which makes the development of skeletal muscle and adipose tissue especially vulnerable to nutritional deficiency [34]. There is some evidence that low birth weight tracks over to a reduced muscle fiber count in older ages, which might underlie the association between lower birth weight and reduced muscle strength [8].

Furthermore, a recent study analyzed with multilevel models the associations of developmental factors (birth weight, growth parameters, motor and cognitive development), father's social class, and adult factors with grip strength at ages 53, 60–64, and 69 years [19]. It is unclear whether developmental factors operate on the rate of decline in grip strength independently or on the same pathways as adult factors. In a prospective, nationally representative British birth cohort, developmental indicators had persisting associations with grip strength from midlife to old age covering 16 years of follow-up. Physical growth, in terms of heavier birth weight and, for men, later puberty and greater weight throughout the growth period, was associated with stronger grip regardless of influences during adulthood. "On time" or early motor development was associated with stronger grip in later life. Childhood cognitive ability was associated with stronger grip and a slower decline in grip strength. In older ages the association of cognition with grip strength became stronger. Higher grip strength and better cognition in old age appear to share underlying developmental indicators. The authors suggested that in old age grip strength changes may increasingly reflect neural aging processes.

The accumulation model focuses on the accumulation and length of exposures instead of the age when they take place. It states that piling up of exposures during the life span influences later health, functioning, and survival. Many different risk factors or extended exposure to one risk factor may lead to the outcome. The dose-response relationship builds incrementally toward the probability of the outcome either in a linear or exponential way. The outcome may represent realized or unrealized features of healthy aging.

To study predictors of survival to extreme old age, an essential element of healthy aging, one should follow up a representative cohort of people studied earlier in life until their death, and this cohort should include members who died at any age as well as long-lived groups of interest. Knowledge on early physiological predictors of exceptional longevity in humans is scarce. It is possible that long-lived people have physiological reserve, which may be observed already in youth or midlife and which makes them less vulnerable to diseases, disability, and mortality in old age.

Centenarians form an appealing research target as their age is a round number and only a small proportion in people born in early years of 1900 reached that age. Centenarian phenotype has been addressed in several earlier studies, but most of the studies are cross-sectional. In summary, centenarians do not form a uniform group of exceptionally vigorous and robust individuals, but rather consist of individuals who can be categorized as frail, normal, or exceptionally high functioning. However, many centenarians appear to have needed less hospital care at given ages than their shorter-lived contemporaries, which supports the idea that living to 100 years and surpassing the current human life expectancy with about 20 years represents a useful endpoint for studies on healthy aging [11].

We studied in the Honolulu Heart Program/Honolulu-Asia Aging Study if grip strength measured at the age of 56–68 years (mean age 62.0 years) predicts remaining length of life up to centenarian years among men born 1900–1909 and followed up to 2009, when all had had a change to reach 100 years of age and their age at death was known. In addition, we assessed whether smoking, physical activity, diagnosed diseases in midlife, and the longevity of parents correlate with length of life. We then examined if these factors underlie the association of grip strength with longevity [30]. The average length of life in this cohort was 82.4 years. Those in the highest tertile of grip strength lived on average 2.2 years longer than those in the lowest third of the grip strength distribution. If the mother had survived to ≥80 years, the survival of offspring was 2.1 years longer compared with if the mother died at age ≤ 60 years. For never vs. ever smokers, the difference was 3.1 years. Absence of chronic conditions in midlife also predicted approximately 3 years longer life. For example, if the participants were in the highest grip strength tertile, their mother had survived ≥80 years, and they had never smoked; the average remaining survival time after baseline was 27.0 years. In contrast, for those in the lowest grip strength tertile, whose mothers died at age ≤ 60 years, and who had smoked, the survival time was 18.1 years. We examined all possible predictor interactions on survival, but none were statistically significant, suggesting that the predictor influences may be additive. The centenarians had 2.5 times the odds of having belonged in the highest third of grip strength in midlife compared with those who died at the age of ≤79 years. The odds for never smoking were almost six times higher, respectively. Centenarians more than twice as often had a mother who survived 80 years or more than those who died at 79 years or younger. Longevity appears in this cohort to be a result of accumulation of good inheritance, health, physiological reserve, and healthy lifestyle choices [30].

The pathway model focuses on the cumulative effect of life events along the developmental trajectories, with early advantage or disadvantage setting a person on a pathway to a later exposure that may induce positive or negative trajectories. The pathway model focuses on the sequential link between multiple exposures. It is also known as the chain-of-risk model since it states that each exposure to a risk factor increases the likelihood of being exposed to another risk factor. Pathways may operate predominantly through biological mechanisms, predominantly through social pathways or through combinations of biological and social pathways. For example, lower childhood socioeconomic situation may increase the risk of passive smoking and lead to repeated respiratory infections, absence from school and lower educational attainment, and subsequent lower socioeconomic position and poorer health.

In a European study, poor health conditions during childhood and lower socioeconomic position at age 10 were associated with worse health in later life assesses as self-rated health, depressive symptoms and activity limitations. In most of the cases, the associations between early-life conditions and later health outcomes remained, although weakened, after adjusting for education and life-course trajectories indicating that there were also direct effects. Among women, between 66% and 75% of the indirect effect of low parental socioeconomic status at childhood on the three considered health outcomes at older age is explained by educational attainment. Childhood socioeconomic position and health can have lasting direct effects on adult health. This indicates that public investments in children are expected to produce long-lasting effects on people's lives. Moreover, the fact that a great part of their influence passes through education means that interventions in the education system may alleviate the harmful consequences of negative experiences during childhood [2]. Favorable childhood socioeconomic status and increases socioeconomic advantages protect against frailty and morbidity, improve recovery rate from health conditions, reduce mortality risk, and increase total life expectancy, and healthy life expectancy. High childhood socioeconomic position may have a stronger protective effect than high adult socioeconomic position indicating the lasting impact of childhood conditions on healthy longevity. Systematic interventions in education, food supply, and availability of medical care for children from impoverished families are crucial. This indicates that public investments in children are expected to produce long-lasting effects on people's lives [5].

The social mobility model is predominantly used to address the effects of socioeconomic exposures. It focuses on the direction of change of an exposure. This model suggests that individual can move in and out of social exposures, such as social classes or income levels. The direction of this change (upward, downward, or non-mobile) determines their later disease risk. In a Swedish study, downward social mobility was linked with an increased risk of myocardial infarction compared with no change in occupation class. Leisure time physical activity and intergeneration social mobility was studied in a systematic review of 13 studies including a total of 44,000 participants from the United Kingdom, Finland, Sweden, Australia, United States, and Brazil. Participants were aged 16–70 years from population-based surveys, occupational cohorts, and primary care registries. Nine of the 13 studies showed that stable high socioeconomic groups reported the highest levels of participation in leisure time physical activity and stable low socioeconomic groups the lowest. Upward and downwardly mobile groups participated in leisure time physical activity at levels between these stable groups [10].

Policies that favor upward social mobility in the population may be useful in promoting public health through more favorable health behaviors. However, the shortcoming of the social mobility model is the challenge of disentangling the effects of the final exposure from the effects of the trajectory leading up to this last exposure [33]. Examples of life course topics studies related to growing old aging are presented in Table 9.1.

Table 9.1 Examples of life course topics relevant to research on growing old

Aspect	Examples of research themes
Biological factors	Examines physiological changes that occur during development and aging
Psychological factors	Studies cognitive changes, mental health issues, and the impact of aging on identity, self-esteem, and emotional Well-being throughout lifespan
Social factors	Explores the influence of social relationships, family dynamics, and community involvement at different ages and how they influence the aging experience
Economic factors	Analyzes the impact of financial stability in earlier life, employment history, and access to resources on elements of quality of life in old age
Cultural factors	Investigates how cultural beliefs and practices influence perceptions of aging and the roles of older adults in society in different time periods
Life transitions	Considers significant life changes (e.g., education, retirement, loss of a spouse, health crises) and their effects on individuals as they age
Health disparities	Examines how socioeconomic status, race, and geography impact health outcomes and access to care through the lifespan and among older adults
Cohort effects	Studies how different generations grow old differently based on historical periods and social contexts, such as generational experiences, technological innovations, or social movements
Resilience and adaptation	Looks at how adaptation to changes and challenges, and recovery from adverse situations changes through lifespan, and how these influences are carried into old age
Intergenerational relationships	Explores the interactions between older adults and younger generations, support and caregiving, shared experiences, parenting and how childhood home atmosphere tracks into wellbeing in old age, and intergenerational influences on health disparities
Historical period	Compares aging trajectories and phenotypes at different historical times such as technological developments, societal changes, crises, generational experiences, and legislation

9.2 Methodological Considerations and Research Examples of Life Course Studies

The essential element of life course studies is longitudinal data where the same people have been followed up from a younger to an older age or until death. Longitudinal studies take a long time to do which may challenge the relevance of the initial study purpose, optimal timing of study waves, minimizing attrition, controlling for competing risks and selective mortality, accounting for historical period effects, complying with data protection and ethical issues, impact and innovativeness of the study, dealing with reduced motivation and increased burden for participating, and financing the study.

9.2.1 The Main Purpose of the Study Evolves

Does the main purpose of the study remain relevant over time? To address growing old, the longest follow-ups available range from midlife to end of life. In practice, it is not possible to start a study with an idea that we will examine how early-life exposures influence outcomes in old age. Probably, initially the study plan was to address outcomes in a few years' time. However, when the study cohort grows old, new opportunities for research may emerge, and some studies worldwide have taken advantage of this.

For example, the initial objectives of the Honolulu Heart Program were to assess risk factors and estimate morbidity and mortality from coronary heart disease and stroke among men of Japanese origin in Honolulu and make comparisons with other populations. The Honolulu Heart Program was initiated in 1965 by the National Heart, Lung and Blood Institute as a prospective study. The participants were American men of Japanese ancestry born in 1900–1919 and living on the island of Oahu in 1965; age at entry 45–68 years; and sample size of 8006. The first examination was completed in 1968 and was followed by the initiation of a second examination that same year. On average 25 years later in 1991, the Honolulu-Asia Aging Study began as a follow-up research. The aim was to assess diseases of old age, with an emphasis on brain aging, dementia, and disability. There were 4768 survivors of the original 8006 men, and 3734 (80% of survivors) participated in the fourth examination with age ranging from 71.0 to 93.0 years (mean, 77.8 years).

This phase of the study created several novel landmark findings about midlife predictors of old age outcomes. One of them assessed grip strength as a predictor of old age disability [29]. At the time, it was known that decreased muscle strength predisposes people to functional limitations and disability. Cross-sectionally, muscle strength is significantly, but not linearly, associated with functional limitations such as walking speed. A minimum level of strength is needed to perform tasks. Conversely, when strength is well above the minimum required level, a reserve capacity exists. Reserve capacity serves as a safety margin that helps prevent functional limitations from developing, e.g., following inactivity and deconditioning associated with surgery or an acute illness. The analyses were limited to those participants who were healthy at baseline. Persons with diseases were excluded. It is unlikely that middle-aged people without severe health problems would have disabilities, and thus it is probable that any observed disabilities 25 years later had emerged after the grip strength assessments. Those in the lowest grip strength tertile had the greatest risk of disability 25 years later, and those in the middle tertile had intermediate risk compared with those in the highest tertile. Muscle strength tracks over the life span: those who had higher grip strength during midlife remained stronger than others in old age. People with greater muscle strength during midlife are at a lower risk of becoming disabled because of their greater reserve of strength regardless of chronic conditions that may develop. Grip strength measurements can identify those at higher risk of physical disability related to low muscle strength. In these persons, exercise interventions aimed at improving strength in all muscle groups could potentially lower the risk of subsequent physical disability. Good grip strength may mark intrinsic vitality that tracks into good functional ability in old age.

Another example of a landmark findings was that intermediate and poor cognitive function increased progressively with increasing level of midlife systolic blood pressure. For every 10-mm Hg increase in systolic blood pressure an increase in risk for intermediate cognitive function of 7% and for poor cognitive function of 9% was observed even after adjustments for multiple confounders laying grounds to controlling of systolic blood pressure levels to reduce the risk for cognitive impairment in old age [20].

Altogether eight waves of assessments were carried after the fourth wave with the latest taking place in 2011–2012 followed up by a mortality surveillance up to 2014, when approximately 97% of the participants had died. There is scarcity of longitudinal studies with several waves of assessments and follow-up until death, which has resulted in using chronological age rather than proximity to death as a point of reference. The final phase of this study was entitled the Hawaii Lifespan and Health Span Study. These data provide unique analytical opportunities to assess patterns and trajectories of functioning prospectively by anchoring the results to how many years before death they take place. In addition, the data allows studies on length of life instead of mortality risk; [23].

Earlier studies have identified two principal patterns of cognitive performance changes preceding death: terminal decline and terminal drop. Terminal decline is characterized by a gradual cognitive decline several years before death. Terminal drop refers to a steep decline in cognitive performance 1–3 years before death. Using the Hawaii Lifespan and Healthspan Study data, Margret et al. [23] found two latent classes of cognitive change. The first class ("maintainers") was characterized by a shallow decline in cognitive test scores, whereas the second class ("decliners") was characterized by accelerated decline in the assessments approaching year of death. The results were in line with the terminal decline hypothesis. The mean change scores for the entire sample were quite stable until about 5 years before death when more noticeable decline was observed. A novel finding was that the first signs of separation in cognitive scores between the "maintainers" and the "decliners" became apparent 15 years before death, which is earlier than was reported before. Among factors that protected from cognitive decline were having a copy of the APOE ε2 allele, a copy of the longevity-associated FOXO3 G allele, and more years of education. This study provided important information about the importance of individual factors for patterns of functional change when growing old.

9.2.2 Attrition, Selective Mortality and Competing Risks in Longitudinal Studies About Growing Old

In longitudinal studies attrition is one of the major methodological problems. Attrition refers to loss of participants during the study. If those who leave the study differ from those who continue participating, the results may become biased, and generalizability may deteriorate. Researchers typically have data available from the earlier waves preceding the dropout. In aging studies, those who stop participation are typically older and more disabled than those who continue, especially if the study participation demands notable efforts such as entering the laboratory or responding to long questionnaires. In population-based studies, socio-demographic variables, such as low educational level, being out of work, and not being married, often predispose to attrition. In addition, unhealthy lifestyle factors, such as smoking, high alcohol consumption, and physical inactivity, are known correlates of non-participation and attrition. Among older people, attrition may also be related to social factors, such as lack of support from spouse or children.

Even if those who stay and those who drop out of a study are similar at baseline, they may be different at the time of follow-up. Researchers seldom have information about how those surviving people who drop out would have responded if they had stayed in the study.

In aging research, selective mortality is an important driver of study attrition. Selective mortality refers to a process whereby more disadvantaged people die at earlier ages than their more advantaged counterparts. This process will change the composition of the longitudinal study cohorts in a non-random way making them seem healthier, more affluent, more educated, and generally better off than they would in the absence of the selection process. For example, health usually declines with increasing age at the individual level. Due to selective mortality, the average health in a study cohort remains stable or possibly even improves as those who are the poorly die out, leaving a healthier group behind. In life course studies, two opposing perspectives on socioeconomic health disparities have been presented. "Cumulative inequality" states that disparities continue to widen with age. "Age-as-leveler" indicates that disparities become smaller in old age. These inconsistencies can be explained by selective mortality. At the individual level, disparities become more extensive supporting cumulative inequality. At cohort level, selective mortality among those who are disadvantaged removes proportionally more frail individuals compared to those who are more advantaged making them more similar at the group level. In aging studies, a wider age range among the participants at the baseline will lead to a larger variation in the mortality hazards across this differently aged group. The higher mortality in the older than younger participants will make the sample gradually resemble the characteristics of the younger sample. As a result, the average age of the cohort increases less than the follow-up time even though all individuals in the sample have aged the same number of years the follow-up took [35].

When study participants are followed up over time, to determine the time to an event of interest, other types of events can also occur. Competing risks are occurrences that prevent the risk of interest from happening during the follow-up and are common in studies where the outcome is not fatal. Competing risk relates to censoring, which refers to a participant leaving the follow-up. For example, in a study examining the risk of hip fracture, a competing risk could be death, because the dead participants are then no more at risk of getting a hip fracture. Because follow-ups do not last indefinitely, end of study surveillance is also a censoring event if it takes place before the outcome of interest happens.

9.2.3 The Response Rates in Complex Health Studies Among Older People

Declining participation rates and increased refusals have been recognized in epidemiological studies at least for 30 years. Epidemiologic aging studies become more and more complex, with sampling taking place over multiple stages; there are several participation rate steps along the path to data collection. This makes it necessary to explicate persons sampled and contacted; the disposition of all those contacted, in terms of eligibility; and those successfully recruited in the study to partial or full completion of data collection. Unfortunately, detailed presentation of participation rates or the numbers of participants involved in every step of a sample construction are sometimes unclear in epidemiologic papers.

A Danish research group studied the associations of the difference in participation rates, design, and interviewer mode with results concerning functioning of centenarians [32]. Participants were birth cohort members born in 1910 (DK-1910) and 1911–1912 (DK-1911). The same assessment instruments were used, but the design was different. Data collection was carried out by trained survey agency interviewers in DK-1910 and trained nurses in DK-1911. Participation rate in DK-1911 (49.8% (251/504)) was lower than in DK-1910 (66.9% (273/408; $P < 0.001$). The proportion of interviews with the participant answering alone or mainly alone was significantly higher in DK-1911 (77%) than in DK-1910 (56%), and the proportion living in a nursing home was significantly lower (44 vs. 54%, respectively). Higher proportions of DK-1911 performed activities of daily living independently compared to DK-1910. Handgrip strength, gait speed, and chair stand test results were almost similar. DK-1911 participants had significantly better 1-year survival than DK-1911 nonparticipants and DK-1910 participants and nonparticipants ($P = 0.001$). These results suggest that lower participation rate may entail selection toward healthier participants in terms of activities of daily living and cognitive functioning.

We examined factors related to taking part in subsequent phases of a study among 75–85-year-old people with four separate data collection steps typically carried out within a 2 weeks' time [28]. First, we sent information about the study through mail and then started data collection by calling the potential participants on the phone to inform them about our study and to collect initial data relevant for nonrespondent analyses. Second, we visited the participants at their home for structured interviews and performance measures of functioning. Third, participants visited research laboratory for physical assessments. Fourth, they were invited to take part in physical activity monitoring over 1 weeks' time using wearable accelerometers. In the first step, the most frequently reported reasons for not participating were lack of time, poor physical or cognitive health, and unwillingness to participate. In total, almost 9% of the phone interviews were answered by proxies. Of those who took part in the at-home assessments, 89.4% also participated in the physical assessments in the research center. In this step, most frequent reasons for nonparticipation were lack of interest, lack of time, health-related issues or fatigue, and obligation to care for someone else. In total, 54.5% of those participating in the physical assessments in the research center also participated in the accelerometry-based physical activity monitoring. In this step, the most frequent reasons for nonparticipation were lack of interest, wish to participate in water-related activities which were prevented when wearing the monitors, and travels. Participation in the accelerometry study phase did not depend on health and functioning, but rather on depressive symptoms and general interest in physical activity. When studying older people, balancing between standardized precision measures of functioning requiring laboratory conditions and minimizing bias due to selective dropout may prove difficult. Flexible recruitment and examination strategies may facilitate participation of older people with diverse health issues in the study.

Participation rates in the different study phases show that older people experiencing health problems are less likely to participate in studies requiring more effort and commitment. This may potentially truncate the distribution of values. Nevertheless, the experiences during the current study suggest that it is feasible to study physical performance at home and in a research center even among those with limitations in health, functioning, and low overall physical activity, including those with early cognitive decline or depressive symptoms. Similarly, it is also feasible to assess time in physical activity of at least moderate intensity and time in upright posture using a questionnaire and accelerometry among people with a large range in health, functioning, and activity. Study purpose and target population are important considerations for decisions of study setting and implementation strategy. The higher precision of the assessment in the research center seemed to compensate for the selective attrition of participants from these assessments when compared to the full sample participating in the home interview [28].

Nonresponse may bias the results if study participation is associated with the research topic of interest, i.e., the exposure, outcome, or relation of interest, which is often the case in health studies of very old people. The difference in the study outcomes between participants and nonparticipants determines the amount of bias present. However, it is worth noting that lower participation rates may not always cause markedly biased results. Comparing data from two identical surveys with participation rates of 61% and 36%, very few significant differences were found across altogether 91 categories. Importantly, in some instances, nonparticipation bias may be higher in surveys with higher participation rates than those with lower participation rates. This is because extreme efforts to increase participation rates may introduce more bias into the study if the added respondents are not representative of all nonrespondents. Additionally, intense recruitment efforts of hesitant participants may be unethical. Since sampling representative populations is needed to illustrating burden of disease for public health planning, collecting minimal data on nonrespondents for comparisons with respondents could provide important information about the representativeness of those responding. However, the institutional review boards may consider this coercion and disagree with the collection of these data [13].

9.3 Period and Cohort Effects on Healthy Aging

Circumstances underlying health may change over time and from one birth cohort to another. It is possible that some cohorts suffer from more risky situations in childhood, start smoking more frequently, exercise less, or eat worse diets than those born earlier or later. However, the general trend has been toward improvement in many European countries. Periods and cohorts and their influences on aging are challenging to distinguish from each other, as all of them contribute to health trends.

Age, period, and cohort represent distinct influences on health changes over time. Periods and cohorts reflect social perspective modifying aging of individuals living in them, while aging refers to changes occurring in individuals when they progress through life span.

Policy makers are often interested in trends. For example, are people physically more or less active than before? Have death rates declined across birth cohorts? Investigating age, period, and cohort patterns can provide new insights about how aging, social changes, and population processes interact with schools, families, and healthcare organizations shaping differences in healthy aging.

An interesting analysis about cohort and period effects comes from Denmark, where between 1975 and 2000 lifespans of women rose, stagnated, and then rose again. The gap between female life expectancy in Denmark vs. Sweden grew to 3.5 years in that period. The influence of the Danish women born 1915–1945 on the overall differences in life expectancy compared with Sweden increased until 1995–1999, by which time, 86% of the total difference between the two countries was attributable to the 1915–1945 generations. The decrease and later increase seen in life expectancy was attributable to specific cohorts born 1915–1945 and not to factors acting on all women alive between 1975 and 2000. Instead it was due to the higher rates of smoking in the interwar generation of Danish women, because the smokers of the interwar generations were dying at younger ages. Thus, the excess mortality decreased with age when the subsequent surviving population consisted of women with healthier lifestyle behaviors or women having factors compensating for unhealthy lifestyle behaviors. All in all, this study showed that the stagnation and the recent increase seen in Danish women's life expectancy mostly could be explained by the increased mortality of the smoking interwar generations of Danish women [21]. This study illustrated a cohort rather than period effect on the life expectancy of Danish women.

9.3.1 Has the Functional Capacity and Health of Older Adults Improved or Declined?

For the question of whether and how the functioning and well-being of older people has changed depends on the approach we take to answering this question. Forty years ago, Professor James Fries introduced the idea of the "compression of morbidity," which provides a useful instrument for debating advances in health among the older population [12]. He proposed that the increased life expectancy would come with less years lived with major diseases, because the same forces that were underlying decreased mortality would also lower the incidence of chronic disease (and disability) and postpone infirmity to higher ages. The opposite idea put forward was that decrease in mortality would result from better survival of people with health problems, resulting in more disease in the population, the process which was termed the failure of success [14]. Subsequently, an idea of dynamic equilibrium was presented. It posits a scenario between these two. According to this hypothesis, the severity and progression of chronic diseases would keep pace with mortality change [22]. At early stages of the progression of a disease, it can be controlled, leading to higher incidence of disease but with diminished consequences, such as disability and death. Since this time, these three scenarios linking the extension of life expectancy at older ages and changes in morbidity and disability—expansion of morbidity, dynamic equilibrium, and compression of morbidity—have provided the hypotheses for much research on trends in health and functioning.

Examining these trends is not simple. Mortality risk has declined even among those aged 100 years. In line with this change, causes of death have changed to chronic diseases with cardiovascular diseases being the leading cause of death among most low-mortality countries. Cardiovascular disease incidence has declined somewhat, but at the same time the prevalence of heart disease has increased from the 1980s through the 1990s and more recently (see [7]). The cardiovascular disease mortality has declined 60% since the 1950s in the United States [24]. This reduction points to the equilibrium model, where the consequences of diseases are less severe including lower mortality risk leading to higher disease prevalence.

The most consistent findings supporting the idea of dynamic equilibrium and coinciding improving functional capacity in the older population have concerned the decreases in the prevalence of functional limitations and reductions in disability at given ages. The functional capacity of individuals of the same age born at different times has been studied for at least ADL and IADL disabilities, mobility, physical capacity, cognitive functions, and psychological well-being. We found substantial improvements in muscle strength, walking speed, cognitive capacity, and emotional well-being between 75- and 80-year-old people examined 28 years apart in 1989–1990 and 2017–2018 [15, 16, 25].

Age-specific functional capacity is likely better now than in past decades up to about 85 years of age, but there is no certainty thereafter. On the contrary, it may be that as a larger proportion of a birth cohort lives to a very old age, the positive trend in more recent cohorts disappears, as longevity becomes less select. However, improvements in cognitive functions; ADL and IADL have been reported also among people aged 90+ years [6]. One of the explanations for the decrease in disability has been that diseases have become less disabling as their progression has been slowed down or even stopped with effective treatments before functional consequences have progressed to disability. This is true of both heart disease and arthritis, two of the most common causes of disability [7]. All in all, compression of morbidity may not hold true, but instead there will be more and more chronic conditions in the older populations, but effective medical treatments have made the consequences of many diseases less grave including lowering gradients of functional decline and reduced mortality rate. In any case, the extension of lifespan means that there are more years of good functional capacity, but at the same time, the absolute number of very old people experiencing functional limitations is higher.

There are also conflicting results. One reason for this may be the difficulty in conducting methodologically completely comparable studies over several decades. In addition, the meaning of specific risk factors change over time. The Survey of Health, Aging and Retirement in Europe (SHARE) suggested that in 2013 people aged 50+ had better cognitive function compared with same-aged persons in 2004–2005, with an average difference of approximately one-third standard deviation. The same level of cognitive function in 2004–2005 at age 50 years was found in 2013 for people who were 8 years older. There was an improvement in cognitive function in all European regions [1]. That study suggested that later-born Europeans had substantially better cognitive functioning than earlier-born cohorts. For physical functioning, improvements were less clear, except for Northern Europe where there was an improvement in ADL and IADL in the oldest age groups. In any case, the extension of lifespan means that there are more years of good functional capacity, but at the same time, the absolute number of very old people experiencing functional limitations is higher.

References

1. Ahrenfeldt LJ, Lindahl-Jacobsen R, Rizzi S, et al. Comparison of cognitive and physical functioning of Europeans in 2004-05 and 2013. Int J Epidemiol. 2018;47:1518–28.
2. Arpino B, Gumà J, Julià A. Early-life conditions and health at older ages: the mediating role of educational attainment, family and employment trajectories. PLoS One. 2018;3:e0195320.
3. Ben-Shlomo Y, Cooper R, Kuh D. The last two decades of life course epidemiology, and its relevance for research on ageing. Int J Epidemiol. 2016a;45:973–88.
4. Ben-Shlomo Y, Cooper R, Kuh D. Life course epidemiology: the last two decades and future directions. Int J Epidemiol. 2016b;45:973–87.
5. Chen Y. Childhood and adult socioeconomic status influence on late-life healthy longevity: evidence from the Chinese longitudinal healthy longevity survey. Front Public Health. 2024;12:1352937.
6. Christensen K, Thinggaard M, Oksuzyan A, et al. Physical and cognitive functioning of people older than 90 years: a comparison of two Danish cohorts born 10 years apart. Lancet. 2013;382:1507–13.
7. Crimmins E, Beltrán-Sánchez H. Mortality and morbidity trends: is there compression of morbidity? J Gerontol. 2011;66B:75–86.
8. Dodds R, Denison HJ, Ntani GN, et al. Baird, birth weight and muscle strength: a systematic review and meta-analysis. J Nutr Health Aging. 2012;16:609–15.
9. Elder GH Jr, Shanahan MJ, Damon W, Lerner RM. The life course and human development. In: Handbook of child psychology, Theoretical models of human development, vol. vol 1. New York: Wiley; 2006. p. 665–715.
10. Elhakeem A, Hardy R, Bann D, et al. Intergenerational social mobility and leisure-time physical activity in adulthood: a systematic review. J Epidemiol Community Health. 2017;71:673–80.
11. Engberg H, Oksuzyan A, Jeune B, et al. Centenarians–a useful model for healthy aging? A 29-year follow-up of hospitalizations among 40,000 Danes born in 1905. Aging Cell. 2009;8:270–6.

12. Fries JF. Aging, natural death, and the compression of morbidity. NEJM. 1980;303:1369–70.
13. Galea S, Tracy M. Participation rates in epidemiologic studies. Ann Epidemiol. 2007;17:643–53.
14. Gruenberg EF. The failures of success. Milbank Mem Fund Q Health Soc. 1977;55:3–24.
15. Kekäläinen T, Koivunen K, Pynnönen K, et al. Cohort differences in depressive symptoms and life satisfaction in 75- and 80-year-olds: a comparison of two cohorts 28 years apart. J Aging Health. 2024;36:3–13.
16. Koivunen K, Sillanpää E, Munukka M, et al. Cohort differences in maximal physical performance: a comparison of 75- and 80-year-old men and women born 28 years apart. J Gerontol Biol Sci Med Sci. 2021;76A:1251–9.
17. Kuh D, Ben-Shlomo Y, Lynch J, et al. Life course epidemiology. J Epidemiol Community Health. 2003;57:778–83.
18. Kuh D, Cooper R, Hardy R, et al. A life course approach to healthy ageing. Oxford: Oxford University Press; 2014.
19. Kuh D, Hardy R, Blodgett JM, et al. Developmental factors associated with decline in grip strength from midlife to old age: a British birth cohort study. BMJ Open. 2019;9:e025755.
20. Launer LJ, Masaki K, Petrovitch H, et al. The association between midlife blood pressure levels and late-life cognitive function. The Honolulu-Asia Aging Study. JAMA. 1995;274:1846–51.
21. Lindahl-Jacobsen R, Rau R, Jeune B. Rise, stagnation, and rise of Danish women's life expectancy. Proc Natl Acad Sci USA. 2016;113:4015–20.
22. Manton KG. Changing concepts of morbidity and mortality in the elderly population. Milbank Mem Fund Q Health Soc. 1982;60:183–244.
23. Margrett JA, Schofield T, Martin P, et al. Novel functional, health, and genetic determinants of cognitive terminal decline: Kuakini Honolulu Heart Program/Honolulu-Asia Aging Study. J Gerontol. 2022;77A:1525–33.
24. Martin SS, Aday AW, Almarzooq ZI, et al. Heart disease and stroke statistics: a report of us and global data from the American Heart Association. Circulation. 2024;149:e347–913.
25. Munukka M, Koivunen K, von Bonsdorff M. Birth cohort differences in cognitive performance in 75- and 80-year-olds: a comparison of two cohorts over 28 years. Aging Clin Exp Res. 2021;33:57–65.
26. Murray GK, Jones PB, Kuh D, Richards M. Infant developmental milestones and subsequent cognitive function. Ann Neurol. 2007;62:128–36.
27. Poranen-Clark T, von Bonsdorff MB, Lahti J, et al. Infant motor development and cognitive performance in early old age: the Helsinki Birth Cohort Study. Age (Dordr). 2015;37:9785.
28. Portegijs E, Karavirta L, Saajanaho M, et al. Assessing physical performance and physical activity in large population-based aging studies: home-based assessments or visits to the research center? BMC Public Health. 2019;19:1570.
29. Rantanen T, Guralnik JM, Foley D, et al. Midlife hand grip strength as a predictor of old age disability. JAMA. 1999;281:558–60.
30. Rantanen T, Masaki K, He Q, et al. Midlife muscle strength and human longevity up to age 100 years: a 44-year prospective study among a decedent cohort. Age (Dordr). 2012;34:563–70.
31. Richards M, Deary IJ. A life course approach to cognitive reserve: a model for cognitive aging and development? Ann Neurol. 2005;58:617–22.
32. Vestergaard S, Andersen-Ranberg K, Skytthe A, et al. Health and function assessments in two adjacent Danish birth cohorts of centenarians: impact of design and methodology. Eur J Ageing. 2015;13:15–23.
33. Wagner C, Carmeli C, Jackisch, et al. Life course epidemiology and public health. Lancet. Public Health. 2024;9:e261–9.
34. Yan X, Zhu MJ, Dodson MV, Du M. Developmental programming of fetal skeletal muscle and adipose tissue development. J Genomics. 2013;1:29–38.
35. Zajacova A, Burgard SA. Healthier, wealthier, and wiser: a demonstration of compositional changes in aging cohorts due to selective mortality. Popul Res Policy Rev. 2013;32:311–24.

Work as Active Aging

10

Abstract

Work refers to an activity involving mental or physical effort done to achieve a purpose or result. Promoting longer working careers is probably the most visible policy action concerning active aging. Currently, proportion of older people working for pay differs extensively between countries. The first studies focusing on changes in well-being around the retirement transition observed significant improvements, but more recently the changes have become less notable possibly due to improvements in the working life during the last decades. Nevertheless, significant policy changes are required to make it possible for people in high-risk profiles to extend their working years. Longitudinal studies show that negative exposures during working life track over to old ages.

Work forms an essential activity of adult life and may take about one-fourth to one-third of the waking hours. It structures passage of time, produces recourses for personal income, and anchors individuals within the social structure. In the context of aging, the dominating questions concerning work include participation in workforce of older people, work ability, retirement, and how work influences old age.

One of the first theories with positive outlook toward aging concerned productive aging introduced by Dr. Robert Butler. Productive aging was used as an umbrella concept covering several activities of older people, such as economic activities, formal and nonformal learning and volunteering, and different types of caregiving. Through these activities, older people contribute to the society and the well-being. The concept helps to support and improve work opportunities and remove barriers for community engagement. The realization of productive aging varies based on opportunities in different countries in terms of the nature and availability of activities considered suitable for older people, cultural and social norms, welfare systems,

T. Rantanen, *Advancing Research on Active Aging and Participation*, https://doi.org/10.1007/978-3-031-94702-5_10

and structural constraints such as laws and regulations concerning upper age limits. The idea of productive aging relates to active aging by emphasizing doing something and optimizing the environment through increasing facilitators and minimizing barriers for the activity.

Employment rates at 55–59, 60–64, 65–69, and 70–74 years are included in the United Nations Economic Commission for Europe (UNECE) Active Aging Index (AAI). Increasing employment rates in older ages is probably the most visible political endeavor concerning active aging (UNECE/European Commission 2015, accessed 18.12.2024). Policies to promote older people to work longer, however, need to create effective public supports which consider the heterogeneity of the older population in terms of their health, capacities, and resources. To restrain social inequalities in old age, working longer needs to be calibrated to the disparity of capacities of older people. The AAI defines active aging as "the situation where people continue to participate in the formal labor market as well as engage in other unpaid productive activities (such as care provision to family members and volunteering) and live healthy, independent and secure lives as they age." This index has been criticized for not considering the older peoples' ability to work nor whether they value working. In addition, having to work in old age or having to put a lot of effort into caring for family members may reflect hardship and lack of social security rather than realizing one's goals and active approach to life.

10.1 Participation in Work Force in Older Ages

In Europe, over the last 10 years, the expected duration of working life increased from 34.7 years in 2013 to 36.9 years in 2023. The Netherlands, Sweden, Denmark, and Estonia had the longest expected duration of working life in 2023, each with more than 40 years. In 2023 in the EU, 10.2% of people who receive an old-age pension were employed. The average retirement age in the EU was 61.3 years, ranging from 58.3 years in Slovenia to 65.7 years in Denmark. 13.0% of people continued to work after receiving their first old-age pension. The highest proportion of people aged 50–74 years who continued to work after starting to receive old age pension were in Northern Europe. Estonia had the highest employment rate and the largest share of persons employed and receiving an old-age pension in the age group of 50–74 years (54.9%). In addition to Estonia, Latvia, Lithuania, and Sweden had relatively high shares of employed people receiving pensions (over 40% of people aged 50 to 74 years). In contrast, some countries had very low shares of employed people with pensions, indicating that pension receipt often marks the end of working life in these countries. In Spain, Greece, and Romania, the share of employed people with pensions was less than 1% among people aged 50–74 and less than 1.5% among people aged 60–74. This suggests that in these countries, pensioners tend to stop working and fully retire, rather than continuing to work in some capacity (https://ec.europa.eu/eurostat/statistics-explained/Duration of working life - statistics - Statistics Explained, accessed 18.12.2024).

10.2 Retirement

Old age retirement refers to stopping working after reaching a given age. The first retirement age was set in Germany in 1889. Otto Von Bismarck drafted the request put forward by the emperor in 1881 as follows "...those who are disabled from work by age and invalidity have a well-grounded claim to care from the state." Originally the age limit was at 70 but was reduced to 65 in 1916. Old age pension was a radical idea, because at that time people needed to work for as long as they survived, except for military personnel and some municipal professions such as police or firefighters in some bigger cities. Following this, more countries began to adopt an official retirement age, such as Britain with the passage of the Old Age Pensions Act in 1908, which set the initial retirement age at 70 before it was reduced to 65 for men and 60 for women with the passage of the National Insurance Act in 1946. The United States adopted an initial retirement age of 65, under the bill of the Social Security Act of 1935. By the mid-twentieth century, almost all countries had adopted a retirement age. The average of statutory retirement age in the 34 countries of the Organisation for Economic Co-operation and Development (OECD) in 2014 was 65 years for men and 63.5 years for women. The trend in most countries is to raise the retirement age. Now, retirement at age 65 years is common in EU Member States. Many countries have decided to raise the retirement age to 67 years. For the main part, the changes in retirement ages are scheduled to take place between 2020 and 2030 (Finnish Centre for Pensions. https://www.etk.fi/en accessed 16.12.2024).

Initially surpassing the age limit of 65 for old age pension was rather rare and retirement applied to only few people. However, by the 1960s and 1970s, life expectancy had risen in many countries to 70 and above, and the number of retired people increased. Increasingly, in the policies of Western countries, the retirement age is being linked to life expectancy. The fact that in many countries more older people are exiting the work force to retirement than younger people are entering the work force has led to an interest in extending working lives for older workers. The traditional view of retirement as an abrupt and one-time exit from the labor market no longer holds true today. The extension of working lives results in an increase in total hours worked and expanded labor supply. Work may have favorable or unfavorable influences on the well-being of aging employees. Detrimental effects on well-being may occur if work is stressful physically or mentally. Potential positive effects on well-being may include providing structure in life, social relationships and support, satisfaction of accomplishments, access to occupational health care, and financial stability. There are contradictory issues concerning working until older ages. Working longer may increase quality of life and living standard. At the same time the feasibility of extending working lives may differ between different jobs, work may also have negative effects, and extending working careers may reflect and even increase social disparities.

The Nordic countries provide an opportunity to study factors associated with working later in a context where older workers are fairly free from compelling financial predicament. Nordic countries represent relatively prosperous societies with extensive welfare services and state and labor market pensions. Consequently, economic constraints less likely prevail the reasons for continuing to work beyond retirement. A large Danish study compared individuals who had retired full time with individuals that were still in the workforce even though they could have retired. They found that individuals who continued in the workforce after their retirement age had greater wealth, were in better health, and were more often men compared to the retirees. The probability that an individual continues in the workforce past retirement age decreases with increasing age, gender (female), years spent in the work force, higher alcohol consumption, and physical activity [22].

Another study using the European Survey of Health, Aging and Retirement in Europe (SHARE) combined information on life histories with information on current retirement. The aim was to understand how working after retirement relates to the previous work history, i.e., number of years in different types of employment, occupational status, and the number of job changes over the work career. The results showed that the larger the share of part-time work or self-employment over the work career, the higher the likelihood to work after retirement. Also, those with high occupational status and flexible careers were particularly likely to work after retirement. Regarding gender, they found that divorced women will likely work after retirement, but only if they did not remarry [1]. The authors concluded that inequalities that develop across the life course continue to play a role after retirement.

Retirement transition is a process that starts years before the actual retirement and depends on retirement intentions. The model of retirement decision-making distinguishes between retirement preferences, retirement intentions, and the act of retiring and describes a process of increasing decisiveness. First, the participants consider the general prospect of retirement or may have an idea of a preferred time for retirement. Subsequently, they proceed to more detailed retirement planning and decisions about timing. Finally, the person retires in line with their articulated plan to retire at a certain age. Whether the retirement intentions translate into actual retirement has not been extensively studied, but there is evidence of a clear link between the retirement intentions and actual retirement. In Finland, retirement plans, as indicated by the intended retirement age, are found to materialize with quite high accuracy. For example, based on the 2008 Quality of Working Life Survey and follow-up register data, almost half of the respondents retired at the exact age they intended to [12]. The 2018 Quality of Working Life Surveys (QWLS) of Statistics Finland was based on a sample of 4110 employees being representative of the working-age employee population in Finland. Concentrating in the age group of 50–62 years predictors of retirement intentions were studied. Gender was not associated with intended retirement age, but age was. The older the respondent, the higher the intended retirement age. Having higher tertiary education correlated with intention to retire later. Somewhat unexpectedly, the intended retirement age did not vary based on socioeconomic status or employment sector. Good perceived work ability was associated with higher intended retirement age and sickness absences with earlier retirement intentions. The family situation was not related to the intended retirement age, except for those who had never married—they intend to retire later. People who led a work-centered life intended to retire later while those who considered hobbies important intended to retire sooner. Somewhat

Table 10.1 A summary of factors related to earlier vs. later retirement

Factor	Earlier retirement	Later retirement
Age	Increased age reduces likelihood of continuing to work	Older individuals report higher intended retirement ages
Gender	Women retire earlier on average	Men are more likely to continue working beyond retirement age
Health	Poor perceived work ability and sickness absences	Better health and perceived work ability
Education	Lower education is related to earlier retirement	Higher tertiary education correlates with later retirement
Economic status	Not related	Economic constraints such as earlier unemployment periods may necessitate continued employment. Also, greater income is associated with continuing work
Employment history	Long careers in physically or mentally stressful jobs	Flexible careers, possibility for part-time work, self-employment, and high status
Marital status	Married individuals retire earlier	Divorced or never-married individuals retire later
Work environment	Layoffs at the workplace	Employer support for older workers' continued employment
Lifestyle factors	Strong focus on hobbies and non-work interests	Work-centered life and satisfaction from work-related accomplishments
Life expectancy trends	Shorter life expectancy in earlier periods led to earlier retirement	Rising life expectancy trends encourage delayed retirement

surprisingly, unemployment experience was associated with higher intended retirement age. In addition to individual factors, also work-related factors underlie retirement intentions. If the respondents felt that their employer supported older workers' continued employment, the intended retirement age was higher. Instead, layoffs at the workplace were conducive to lower intended retirement age [12].

In Finland, of 20–64-year-old people, over 70% believe that they can continue working in their current profession until statutory retirement age. Of the 65–75-year-old people, 55% consider themselves fully able to work (https://repo.thl.fi/sites/tervesuomi/ilmioraportit_2023/tyokyky.html, accessed 18.12.2024) (Table 10.1).

10.3 Work and Well-Being After Retirement

Retirement from regular work changes the daily exposure to different positive and negative psychological, social, and physiological stress factors and may thus also influence the well-being. However, only few studies concerning work and occupational health have follow-ups extending to over the retirement transition and up to old age. One of the landmark studies of the transition between professionally active life and retirement on determinants of early aging and of the persistence of long-term effects of occupational exposures is called the GAZEL Cohort Study, which was launched in January 1989 among Électricité de France-Gaz de France (EDF-GDF) workers. In 1989, the original cohort comprised 20,625 participants (15,011 male employees aged 40–50 years and 5614 women between 35 and 50 years old). Follow-up is still ongoing and continuous and includes data collection on health status, lifestyle, and socioeconomic and occupational factors from various sources. A mailed questionnaire is sent to the participants each year, and data are extracted regularly from the files of the personnel and medical departments of EDF-GDF and from national registers [5]. The GAZEL is an epidemiological laboratory in the sense that it is not optimized for any specific research questions but instead it is open to researchers' proposals.

The GAZEL study includes extensive information about of work characteristics and exposures including occupational grade, income, and commuting time. This provides an opportunity to study how work characteristics relate to different indicators of health and health behavior. Physical and mental stress factors included information on working with the public, outdoor work, night work, regular work hours, on-call work, standing work posture, hard work posture, handling heavy loads, exposure to vibrations, working with a computer screen, working in the cold, working in the heat, exposure to noise, work involving specific risks, and work administratively classified as unhealthy. In addition, physically demanding work, nerve-wracking work, and satisfactory work, decision latitude, psychological demands, social support, extrinsic effort, and reward at work were queried. Information on constant strain, effort/reward imbalance, and overcommitment were included as well. For each worker, working conditions were estimated as the sum of the scores for all indicators divided by the number of available indicators [11].

In a comprehensive analysis on the association of work exposures and the cardiovascular disease risk factors, the authors found that several of the included work stress factors predicted incident cardiovascular risk factors, such as alcohol consumption, physical inactivity, obesity, and sleep disturbances. They used the 1989 data as baseline with average follow-ups ranging between 3 and almost 12 years [11].

- Increased risk of non-moderate alcohol consumption was more common among those in higher occupational grade, higher decision latitude, more social support at work, and presence of constant strain.
- Physical inactivity was more common among those with lower monthly income and who reported indicators of physically demanding work.
- Risk of obesity correlated with altogether 19 indicators of working conditions. Risk was increased by low occupation grade and income, working with public, night work, outdoor work, work on call, indicators of physically heavy work, working in cold or heat, exposure to noise, and work including specific risks or unhealthy element. More social support at work, rewards, and absence of effort reward imbalance protected from obesity.

- Sleep complaints were predicted by 22 working conditions with negative features increasing the risk and positive conditions (rewards, higher decision latitude, and satisfactory work) decreasing the risk. Findings for risk of depression were largely parallel to sleep complaints.

These results suggest the existence of close relationships between a poor work environment and a higher risk of developing obesity, sleep complaints, or depression. The mechanisms by which work environment might influence these risk factors are still a matter of debate. It is evident that work-related risk factors contribute to increased CVD risk through CVD risk factors at the time when workers are exposed to poor working conditions in their work. However, the influences of obesity, sleep disturbances, non-moderate alcohol consumption, and physical inactivity may track over years after retirement and that way they may predict development of other risk factors and future decline in health even when work risk factors are not anymore present.

Taking advantage of annually repeated assessments, several analyses have been conducted on changes in health and health-related behaviors around retirement in the GAZEL study. Retirement from work reduced prevalence of many negative health corollaries. The authors assessed general perceived health with an eight-category standard Likert scale question repeated in the same way every year. Four poorest categories were considered as suboptimal health. The year before retirement, suboptimal health was reported by 19.2% and the year after retirement by 14.3% of the participants. High psychological and physical work demands were related to a larger increase in prevalence of suboptimum health before retirement and increased benefit around retirement. High job satisfaction was associated with a significantly slower increase in the prevalence of suboptimum health before retirement and less benefit from retirement, whereas those with low job satisfaction benefited the most from retirement. The authors created a high risk and a low risk profile of work-related factors and studied their trajectories around retirement. The high-risk profile included low occupational grade, high work demands, and low work satisfaction. The low-risk profile consisted of high occupational grade, low physical and psychological work demands, and high job satisfaction. In the low-risk scenario, no retirement-related improvements in health were noted, and the prevalence of suboptimal health remained under 5% throughout the 14-year follow-up around the year of retirement. In the high-risk scenario, the estimated prevalence of suboptimal health decreased from approximately 30% to approximately 20% around the retirement, but after a few years, it started to increase again [21]. Results in line with these were observed also for sleep disturbances, headache, depression, and fatigue [5]. Also, life satisfaction, a cognitive component of psychological well-being, may improve around the retirement transition. In a Finnish study, life satisfaction before retirement differed by occupational categories with higher life satisfaction among those in high-skill level than among those in low-skill level occupations. Total life satisfaction score improved among the entire study population during the retirement transition and remained stable thereafter [15]. The improvement was greater among women versus men, among those with suboptimal health before retirement vs. those who had good health and those who had no spouse vs. those who had a retired or working spouse.

10.4 Health Behaviors and Activities Around Retirement

When people disengage from work, they will have more time to spend in new ways. Retirement has the potential to lead to changes in various activities which may influence health and well-being in a positive way. However, it is also possible that stopping working does not dispose of the long-term bearings of work on behaviors and activities. The Finnish Retirement and Aging (FIREA) Study was set up to follow up changes in health behavioral and cardiometabolic risk factors across retirement transition and to examine the long-term consequences of work and retirement on health and functioning with advancing age [17]. Public sector workers whose estimated statutory retirement date was in 2014–2019 were invited to participate by sending them a questionnaire 18 months prior to their estimated retirement date. In the first phase of the FIREA Study, participants were followed up with annual surveys, accelerometer, and clinical measurements during retirement transition into post-retirement years. The FIREA survey cohort includes 6783 participants, of which 908 belong also to the physical activity substudy and 290 to the clinical substudy.

The FIREA results suggested that daily sedentary time was 8 h 10 min in women and 9 h 49 min in men before retirement. Considering all measurement days before and after retirement, daily sedentary time increased in women by 29 min after retirement. Especially women retiring from manual occupations showed a marked increase in sedentary time (63 min). When only non-working days before retirement were considered, increase in daily sedentary time among women was less marked (16 min). Among men, daily sedentary time did not change in retirement transition (−7 min; [18]). Subsequently, the authors studied different intensities of physical activity behavior in an analysis where data were pooled and harmonized with the Swedish Retirement Study. Over the retirement transition, total physical activity decreased 11 min per day. Moderate to vigorous physical activity remained stable and sedentary time did not change. Higher physical activity was cross-sectionally associated with better self-rated health, but no significant associations were observed between changes in the physical activity variables during retirement transition and self-rated health at postretirement follow-ups [4]. However, increasing physical activity at the expense of passive behaviors was associated with a better lipid profile [19]. Physical activity was also observed to coincide with trajectories of physical functioning over the retirement transition. High or fluctuating physical activity trajectories often included participants with stable high physical functioning, while coincident decreasing functioning and stable low activity formed an observed trajectory also characterized by obesity, high-risk use of alcohol, and being a single woman [10].

Table 10.2 Summary of sequel to retirement in higher and lower grade occupations

Higher-grade occupations	Lower grade occupations
Less drastic health or behavioral changes post-retirement because of better baseline conditions, higher job satisfaction, and greater financial security. Often a desire to continue working albeit in a different context than before retirement	Retirement is often a more transformative period bringing relief from negative work environments and improvements in health and Well-being. However, these benefits may be tempered by increased sedentary behavior; financial challenges, sometimes with increased alcohol consumption; and potential long-term health declines

The Finnish results with retirement transition dating from some 20 years later than that of the GAZEL study indicate more modest benefits of retirement on different health-related indicators. Parallel findings were observed in preretirement job characteristics tracking over to post-retirement period. It is possible that work conditions have improved over these 20 years making retirement transition less momentous. The findings that physical activity decreased after retirement are somewhat surprising considering that after retirement, there is more time that people may use for activities other than work. One explanation may be that going to and coming from work as well as work itself may require active transportation. Work may include changing of body positions and walking to different work workstations accumulating physical activity through the workday. It is also worth noting that the GAZEL and FIREA cohorts differ in terms of gender distribution and occupations.

The continuity theory suggests that after retirement, people are prone to replace work with other meaningful activities in line with their value system and preferences. This suggests that retirement transition might provide a fruitful window of opportunity for adopting new positive activities and health enhancing habits especially for those who have endured negative working conditions and who may receive more time and energy for new activities (see Table 10.2). However, if hard work has taken most of the energy out of a person, the threshold to start new activities may be high. It appears that people do not spontaneously adopt a new way of life after retirement. Rather it appears that many might benefit from more systematic support for initiating new activities during the retirement transition.

10.5 Work Exposures and Old Age Disability and Activity

Even though the strain of work is withdrawn during the retirement transition, economic issues, customary health behaviors, health problems, or customary approach to life activities may still track over for several years extending into older ages. The Finnish Longitudinal Study of Municipal Employees (FLAME) is a longitudinal study on Finnish municipal workers conducted at the Finnish Institute of Occupational Health from 1981 to 2009. This study provides unique opportunities to study long-term consequences of different occupational influences present in midlife on health in older ages. In 1981, a total of 6257 municipal workers (85.2% of those targeted) born in 1923 to 1935 and aged 44–58 years in different areas of

Finland responded to a postal questionnaire. Inclusion criteria were having been working as a municipal worker for at least 5 years. Follow-up data were collected with postal questionnaires in 1985 ($n = 5556$), 1992 ($n = 4534$), 1997 ($n = 3815$), and 2009 ($n = 3093$). The topics studied in the questionnaire survey include work demands, work ability, health, lifestyle, and leisure time activities. The register data on work disability pension, retirement, and causes of death for the year 1981–2013 are also available. This study differs from the GAZEL and FIREA studies by extending into older ages; the respondents were 72 to 86 years old at the time of the latest follow-up.

The long follow-up of FLAME provided an opportunity study whether the expected work-related stress relief resulting from retirement might even out health differences way past retirement [14]. Midlife job profiles mainly linked with physically heavy work were strong predictors of disability in later life. In FLAME, work-related stress symptoms were assessed with postal questionnaires at baseline in 1981 and 4 years later on. At those waves, the participants were asked to consider their responses from the point of view of health, work ability, and working conditions. The stress questionnaire was constructed based on the best knowledge available in the late 1970s and early 1980s when the study was launched [9]. Briefly, four stress profiles were created.

- *Negative reactions to work and depressiveness* included self-reported urge to stay home instead of going to work, lack of energy and vitality, inability to enjoy daily life, inclination to be off work without reason, general reluctance, gloomy outlook for the future, and depression.
- *Perceived decrease in cognition* included difficulty remembering, remembering that requires effort, and blackouts.
- *Sleep disturbances* included difficulty falling asleep, several awakenings during the night, and difficulty falling asleep after awakenings.
- *Somatic symptoms* included chest pain, stomachache, and dizziness.

Persons with a stress score in the lowest tertile in 1981 and 1985 were categorized as having *no stress*. Those whose score was in the highest tertile in both 1981 and 1985 were categorized as having *constant stress*, while all others were considered to have *occasional stress*. We saw a clear gradient of increasing disability severity in old age for increasing intensity of midlife stress symptoms. In comparison with the participants with no stress symptoms, the extensively adjusted left-censored and logistic regression models showed that in old age, disability scores were almost 2–4 units higher, and risk for mobility limitation was 2–3 times higher for those with constant stress symptoms in midlife. We concluded that among occupationally active 44- to 58-year-old men and women, perceived stress symptoms in midlife correlated with disability 28 years later [9]. Stress symptoms may be the first signs of decompensation of individual functioning relative to environmental demands, which may later manifest in disabilities. Our results did not support the idea that the relief from work as such would even out the health trajectories in older ages between those with higher vs. lower work-related stress.

Several studies have consistently reported that for future trajectories of health and mobility, physically demanding work may have negative influences in contrast to physical activity during leisure which is linked to beneficial influences on future functioning. FLAME provided us an opportunity to study whether the expected positive influence of midlife leisure time physical activity might counteract the expected negative influence of midlife occupational physical activity on mobility trajectories. Based on baseline responses, three leisure time physical activity and three occupational physical activity categories were created: light, moderate, or vigorous. Mobility limitations were assessed using a self-reported questionnaire in 1985, 1992, 1997, and 2009. The latest available measure of mobility was used in the analyses. A summary score of mobility was calculated, ranging from zero (no difficulty in any activity) to eight (at least some difficulties in all included mobility tasks). We adjusted the models for the competing risk of mortality and for several potential baseline covariates. We found, first, a clear gradient of increased risk of mobility limitation for increasing occupational activity, i.e., those doing heavy work were more likely to develop more mobility limitations. Participants with vigorous occupational activity in midlife had on average a 23% higher risk and those with moderate occupational activity an 18% higher risk (model adjusted for age, sex, and the other type of PA) for a unit increase in mobility limitation in old age than those with light occupational activity. Leisure time physical activity showed opposite results. The risk of mobility limitations was 31% lower with vigorous leisure time physical activity and 7% lower with moderate leisure time physical activity than with inactivity in the model adjusted for age, sex, and the other type of physical activity. To study the combined effects of occupational and leisure time activity on developing mobility limitations, we set the expected best-case scenario, i.e., those with light occupational activity and vigorous leisure physical activity as the reference. The highest the risk for developing mobility limitations (approximately 50% higher per unit increase) was observed for those with vigorous occupational activity and physically inactive leisure. However, risk of mobility limitations among those with high leisure and occupational physical activity did not differ from the reference. We concluded that negative influences of occupational physical activity may be counteracted with leisure occupation activity [6].

The positive effects of physical activity stem from increased energy expenditure and relate to a lower risk of metabolic diseases (type 2 diabetes mellitus) and atherosclerotic diseases (cardio- and cerebrovascular and peripheral arterial disease). Also, many occupational activities reach or exceed the level of moderate intensity and people in physically heavy jobs may receive similar benefits. However, negative effects of occupational activity are typically associated with the biomechanical loads of lifting, twisting, squatting, and bending. These movements—if used as exercise in controlled and structured settings—can have beneficial effects on the musculoskeletal system, but they can also increase the risk of musculoskeletal symptoms and diseases, especially if awkward postures, heavy loads, vibration, and repetitive or continuous strains are involved. Likely, such movements occur throughout a full working day making the load much higher in individuals with heavy work that than in those with vigorous leisure time physical activity. Young manual workers may to be able to benefit from high biomechanical loads during work by increased physical fitness, but there may be a reversal of the positive effect of heavy work on fitness with advancing age [6].

The FLAME was in the key role in innovating the work ability index, which is an instrument used in clinical occupational health and research to assess work ability during health examinations and workplace surveys. The development of the work ability index started in Finland in the 1990s when there were significant challenges of work force aging. The employment rates of older workers (55+) were around 40%, and early retirement and work disability rates were rather common in many European countries with only minority of workers reaching the mandatory retirement age [8]. The index is based on self-reported answers to a series of questions on the demands of work, the worker's health status, and resources. The questionnaire is self-administered and can be filled in, for example, before an interview with an occupational health professional. The items are as follows: current work ability compared with lifetime best, work ability in relation to the demands of the job, number of current diseases diagnosed by a physician, estimated work impairment due to diseases, sick leave during the past year (12 months), own prognosis of work ability 2 years from now, and mental resources [7].

The work ability index has been found to predict work disability, retirement, and mortality. We found that work ability in midlife predicted decline in health and functioning among men and women during the 28-year follow-up even after adjustment for health and lifestyle factors. The risks showed similar gradients among blue- and white-collar employees, but risk of death was generally higher among blue-collar employees. The fact that work ability in midlife predicted disability almost three decades later despite the competing risk of death indicates that work ability may be considered as an early predictor of the risk of disability in old age [20]. To improve work ability requires efforts and agreement from the workers, the managers, and the employers. The work ability is a result of the interactions of four tiers having complex interactions: (1) health and functional capacity; (2) competence, work experience, and learning; (3) values, attitudes, and motivation; and (4) work, work environment, work community, and management (Fig. 10.1). The interactions of human resources and work are dynamic and change over time. Because work ability is constituted as relationships that change over the years, the results of interventions aiming to promote work ability have not been consistent. A meta-analysis of 17 randomized control trials showed the small positive influences on work ability may be gained by workplace interventions [13]. A poor balance between the elements of work ability decreases the work ability. This imbalance may underlie the decrease in work ability with increasing age. Most studies show that that the imbalance stems from problems in work organization and management together with the decline of workers' personal resources due to aging. The promotion of work ability through developing work management and in the same time supporting workers' personal resources form a potential key area for policies aiming to lengthen work careers and increase employment participation of older people [8].

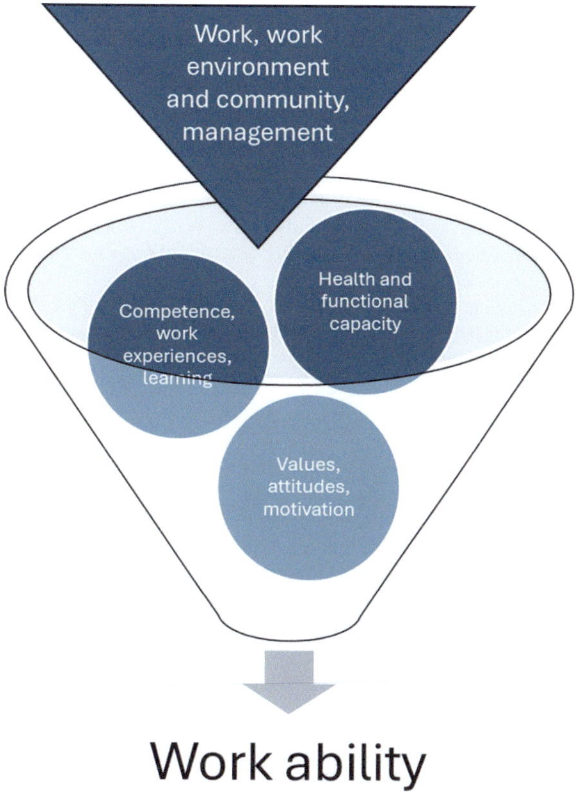

Fig. 10.1 The interacting elements of work ability. This figure is inspired by the work ability house model launched by Juhani Ilmarinen [8]. Management and leadership skills have the strongest effect on work ability. Factors like appreciation, trust, fair treatment, and support effect workplace well-being. Sustainable balance between factors of work and personal resources creates good work ability

The findings from FLAME suggest that the health and well-being of individuals in physically strenuous jobs and those with decreased work ability is markedly worse among workers approaching retirement. Subsequent to retirement some improvement in well-being is observed, which may later vanish. Several work-related risk factors predicted poorer functioning and health years after retirement which underlines the need to better the work life realities. Most Western countries are aiming to increase the economically active proportion of the population by pushing retirement age upward. This is not feasible unless serious consideration is given to the restructuring of work to enable older workers to remain economically active without compromising their present and future health.

References

1. Dingemans E, Möhring K. A life course perspective on working after retirement: what role does the work history play? Adv Life Course Res. 2019;39:23–33.
2. Duration of working life – statistics – European Commission. https://ec.europa.euindex.php. Accessed 18.12.2024. n.d.
3. Finnish Centre for Pensions. https://www.etk.fi/en. Accessed 16.12.2024 n.d.

4. Fröberg A, Sacco L, Suorsa K, et al. Changes in accelerometer-measured physical activity and sedentary time across retirement transition as a predictor of self-rated health. J Phys Act Health. 2024;21:778–86.
5. Goldberg M, Leclerc A, Zins M. Cohort profile update: the GAZEL cohort study. Int J Epidemiol. 2015;44:77–77g.
6. Hinrichs T, von Bonsdorff MB, Törmäkangas T, et al. Inverse effects of midlife occupational and leisure time physical activity on mobility limitation in old age–a 28-year prospective follow-up study. J Am Geriatr Soc. 2014;62:812–20.
7. Ilmarinen J. The Work Ability Index (WAI). Occup Med. 2007;57:160.
8. Ilmarinen J. From work ability research to implementation. Int J Environ Res Public Health. 2019;16:2882.
9. Kulmala J, von Bonsdorff MB, Stenholm S, et al. Perceived stress symptoms in midlife predict disability in old age: a 28-year prospective cohort study. J Gerontol A Biol Sci Med Sci. 2013;68:984–91.
10. Lintuaho R, Saltychev M, Pentti J, et al. Concurrent changes in physical activity and physical functioning during retirement transition-a multi-trajectory analysis. PLoS One. 2023;18:e0293506.
11. Meneton P, Lemogne C, Herquelot E, et al. Primary cardiovascular disease risk factors predicted by poor working conditions in the GAZEL cohort. Am J Epidemiol. 2017;186:815–23.
12. Nivalainen S. Retirement intentions and increase in statutory retirement age: 2017 pension reform and intended retirement age in Finland. J Aging Soc Policy. 2023;36:1115–36.
13. Oakman J, Neupane S, Proper KI, et al. Work place interventions to improve work ability: a systematic review and meta-analysis of their effectiveness. Scand J Work Environ Health. 2018;44:134–46.
14. Prakash KC, Neupane S, Leino-Arjas P, et al. Midlife job profiles and disabilities in later life: a 28-year follow-up of municipal employees in Finland. Int Arch Occup Environ Health. 2016;89:997–1007.
15. Prakash KC, Virtanen M, Törmälehto S, et al. Changes in life satisfaction during the transition to retirement: findings from the FIREA cohort study. Eur J Ageing. 2022;19:1587–99.
16. Social Security History. https://www.ssa.gov/history/ottob.html. Accessed 16.1.2025 n.d.
17. Stenholm S, Suorsa K, Leskinen T, et al. Finnish retirement and aging study: a prospective cohort study. BMJ Open. 2023;13:e076976.
18. Suorsa K, Pulakka A, Leskinen T, et al. Objectively measured sedentary time before and after transition to retirement: the Finnish retirement and aging study. J Gerontol A Biol Sci Med Sci. 2020;75:1737–43.
19. Suorsa K, Leskinen T, Gupta N, et al. Longitudinal associations between 24-h movement behaviors and Cardiometabolic biomarkers: a natural experiment over retirement. Med Sci Sports Exerc. 2024;56:1297–306.
20. von Bonsdorff MB, Seitsamo J, Ilmarinen J, et al. Work ability in midlife as a predictor of mortality and disability in later life: a 28-year prospective follow-up study. CMAJ. 2011;183:E235–42.
21. Westerlund H, Kivimäki M, Singh-Manoux A, et al. Self-rated health before and after retirement in France (GAZEL): a cohort study. Lancet. 2009;374:1889–96.
22. Zaccagni S, Sigsgaard AM, Vrangbaek K, et al. Who continues to work after retirement age? BMC Public Health. 2024;24:692.

Appendix: The University of Jyväskylä Active Aging Scale

Assessment Notes for the University of Jyvaskyla Active Aging Scale (UJACAS)

Active aging is one of the most broadly used terms of positive gerontology. World Health Organization (WHO) defined active aging as a policy goal in 2002 as follows: "Active aging is the process of optimizing opportunities for health, participation and security in order to enhance quality of life as people age" (World Health Organization 2002). The same document also states: "these policies and programmes should be based on the rights, needs, preferences and capacities of older people." The idea was to set a goal for societies. The WHO active aging definition can be used to guide, e.g., comparison of countries regarding how age-friendly they are.

To make it possible to study active aging of individual people, we suggest the following definition: *The striving for elements of well-being through activities relating to a person's goals, functional capacities, and opportunities.* This definition encompasses four central aspects in the active aging of individuals: their goals (what they want to do), their functional capacity (what they are able to do), their autonomy (perceived opportunities to do the valued activities), and their activities (what they actually do). The expected outcome of active aging is promotion of well-being.

About UJACAS

The UJACAS is a quantitative scale for assessing active aging among older people. However, we have not provided any exact age limits for older people. The UJACAS has 17 items with four dimension (goals, ability, opportunity, and activity), and the score ranges between 0 and 272. Response options are worded to suit the item and scored from zero (lowest, e.g., least active) to four (highest, e.g., most active). Scores are computed by summing the scores of the individual items

T. Rantanen, *Advancing Research on Active Aging and Participation*, https://doi.org/10.1007/978-3-031-94702-5

(response option range 0–4) of each dimension to form a subscale and of the total questionnaire to form the total score. A maximum of two missing items is allowed for each subscale and eight for the total sum score. To correct for missing items, we used the following formulas: (sum score/number of items responded to) * number of items offered. The number of items offered is 17 for each subscale and 68 for the total scale.

The psychometric and item properties are good and the scale assesses a unidimensional latent construct of active aging.

Who should use UJACAS?

UJACAS can be used in research and practice among older people. It measures individuals' strive for activity in essential life areas. It describes the active agency of older people, i.e., their initiative to act independently and to make their own free choices. In gerontology, UJACAS provides us knowledge about positive aspects of aging. It can also be used to assess the effectiveness of various interventions aiming to promote active aging.

Scale Development

Developing the scale was a multifaceted process in which we placed high importance on participant feedback and on quantitatively analyzing item properties. We started with a draft scale produced by an expert panel, collected a pilot dataset for item response analyses and for testing validity, conducted two focus group discussions, and tested the scale's reliability in a test-retest study.

Psychometric Properties

The UJACAS questionnaire comprises 17 items including four dimensions yielding four subscores. The minimum total score is zero and the maximum 272. We validated the UJACAS scores against other indicators of activity and well-being and an examination by an occupational therapist. All the indicators of validity and reliability are good. The item analyses showed that the UJACAS subscores capture an underlying single construct that reflects active aging and hence the total score describes active aging in a condensed form.

Limitations

One limitation is that UJACAS may generate socially desirable answers, because active approach to life is generally highly valued in Western societies. Another limitation is that the scale has been developed in the Northern European context and using it in different cultures may require further validation.

Strengths

While we developed the UJACAS we emphasized feedback from participants. User involvement in aging research has benefits. First of all, older people should be able to influence the research that is being conducted on them. Second of all, the chance of producing findings of relevance for the well-being of older people is likely to be higher if they have been invited to contribute their own understandings of the issue. Other strengths include conceptual research and novel definition of active aging that preceded the scale development and the multi-phased development process.

Copyright

The copyright owner of the scale is University of Jyvaskyla.

Administration and Cost

There is no charge to use UJACAS. To get access to the full scale, we ask you to register as an UJACAS user. In the registration form, please let us know whether you intend to translate the UJACAS into a different language. The scale is already available in Finnish, Swedish, and English. We ask you to give your contact information and a brief description of your study and to agree to the terms of using the scale. Please keep track of possible updates of the scale that we will announce at this website.

Collaborators translating UJACAS are requested to send the translated version to the UJACAS research group (details below). Translations of the UJACAS will be posted on the website that distributes UJACAS for use by other researchers and practitioners.

On Behalf of the UJACAS Research Group

Taina Rantanen, Professor of Gerontology and Public Health, Gerontology Research Center, University of Jyvaskyla, PO Box 35, Fi-40014 University of Jyvaskyla, taina.rantanen@jyu.fi

Terms of Use

All costs of reproducing the scale or administering it in a study are the responsibility of the user. The test may be used in an interview or as a mailed questionnaire. No further training is required for administering the scale. The original manuscript describing the scale should be cited as follows: (Rantanen T, Portegijs E, Kokko K, Rantakokko M, Törmäkangas T, Saajanaho M. Developing an Assessment Method of Active Aging: University of Jyvaskyla Active Aging Scale. Journal of Aging and Health 2019; 31:1002-1024. https://doi.org/10.1177/0898264317750449).

Thank you!

Answer each statement (1-17)

	WILL TO ACT	ABILITY TO ACT	POSSIBILITY TO ACT	FREQUENCY OF DOING
	How strongly have you wanted to do the following things **during the past four weeks**?	Bearing in mind **your state of health and your capacity**, have you or would you have been able to do the following things **during the past four weeks**?	Thinking about **your life in general**, how have you experienced your possibilities to do the following things **during the past four weeks**?	How often have you done the following things **during the past four weeks**?
1	**I have wanted to do crafting, DIY or other pastimes requiring manual skills** 4. Very strongly 3. Fairly strongly 2. To some extent 1. Only a little 0. Not at all	**I have or would have been able to do crafting, DIY or other pastimes requiring manual skills** 4. Yes, without any difficulty 3. Yes, but with some difficulty 2. Yes, but with a lot of difficulty 1. Not without help from another person 0. Not even with help	**My possibilities to do crafting, DIY or other pastimes requiring manual skills have been** 4. Very good 3. Rather good 2. Moderate 1. Limited 0. It has not been possible	**I have done crafting, DIY or other pastimes requiring manual skills** 4. Daily or almost daily 3. 2-4 times a week 2. About once a week 1. Less than once a week 0. Not at all
2	**I have wanted to draw, sing or play a musical instrument, write or practice some other artistic pursuit** 4. Very strongly 3. Fairly strongly 2. To some extent 1. Only a little 0. Not at all	**I have or would have been able to draw, sing or play a musical instrument, write or practise some other artistic pursuit** 4. Yes, without any difficulty 3. Yes, but with some difficulty 2. Yes, but with a lot of difficulty 1. Not without help from another person 0. Not even with help	**My possibilities to draw, sing or play a musical instrument, write or practise some other artistic pursuit have been** 4. Very good 3. Rather good 2. Moderate 1. Limited 0. It has not been possible	**I have drawn, sung or played a musical instrument, written or practiced some other artistic pursuit** 4. Daily or almost daily 3. 2-4 times a week 2. About once a week 1. Less than once a week 0. Not at all
3	**I have wanted to take part in various events or activities to do with studying or with clubs or associations** 4. Very strongly 3. Fairly strongly 2. To some extent 1. Only a little 0. Not at all	**I have or would have been able to take part in various events or activities to do with studying or with clubs or associations** 4. Yes, without any difficulty 3. Yes, but with some difficulty 2. Yes, but with a lot of difficulty 1. Not without help from another person 0. Not even with help	**My possibilities to take part in various events or activities to do with studying or with clubs or associations have been** 4. Very good 3. Rather good 2. Moderate 1. Limited 0. It has not been possible	**I have taken part in various events or activities to do with studying or with clubs or associations** 4. Daily or almost daily 3. 2-4 times a week 2. About once a week 1. Less than once a week 0. Not at all
4	**I have wanted to go outside and enjoy the nature** 4. Very strongly 3. Fairly strongly 2. To some extent 1. Only a little 0. Not at all	**I have or would have been able to go outside and enjoy the nature** 4. Yes, without any difficulty 3. Yes, but with some difficulty 2. Yes, but with a lot of difficulty 1. Not without help from another person 0. Not even with help	**My possibilities to go outside and enjoy the nature have been** 4. Very good 3. Rather good 2. Moderate 1. Limited 0. It has not been possible	**I have gone outside and enjoyed the nature** 4. Daily or almost daily 3. 2-4 times a week 2. About once a week 1. Less than once a week 0. Not at all

Answer each statement (1-17)

	WILL TO ACT How strongly have you wanted to do the following things **during the past four weeks**?	ABILITY TO ACT Bearing in mind **your state of health and your capacity**, have you or would you have been able to do the following things **during the past four weeks**?	POSSIBILITY TO ACT Thinking about **your life in general**, how have you experienced your possibilities to do the following things **during the past four weeks**?	FREQUENCY OF DOING How often have you done the following things **during the past four weeks**?
5	**I have wanted to practice keeping physically fit** 4. Very strongly 3. Fairly strongly 2. To some extent 1. Only a little 0. Not at all	**I have or would have been able to practice keeping physically fit** 4. Yes, without any difficulty 3. Yes, but with some difficulty 2. Yes, but with a lot of difficulty 1. Not without help from another person 0. Not even with help	**My possibilities to practice keeping physically fit have been** 4. Very good 3. Rather good 2. Moderate 1. Limited 0. It has not been possible	**I have practiced keeping physically fit** 4. Daily or almost daily 3. 2-4 times a week 2. About once a week 1. Less than once a week 0. Not at all
6	**I have wanted to make an effort to exercise my mind or memory** 4. Very strongly 3. Fairly strongly 2. To some extent 1. Only a little 0. Not at all	**I have or would have been able to make an effort to exercise my mind or memory** 4. Yes, without any difficulty 3. Yes, but with some difficulty 2. Yes, but with a lot of difficulty 1. Not without help from another person 0. Not even with help	**My possibilities to make an effort to exercise my mind or memory have been** 4. Very good 3. Rather good 2. Moderate 1. Limited 0. It has not been possible	**I have made an effort to exercise my mind or memory** 4. Daily or almost daily 3. 2-4 times a week 2. About once a week 1. Less than once a week 0. Not at all
7	**I have wanted to use a computer or a pad** 4. Very strongly 3. Fairly strongly 2. To some extent 1. Only a little 0. Not at all	**I have or would have been able to use a computer or a pad** 4. Yes, without any difficulty 3. Yes, but with some difficulty 2. Yes, but with a lot of difficulty 1. Not without help from another person 0. Not even with help	**My possibilities to use a computer or a pad have been** 4. Very good 3. Rather good 2. Moderate 1. Limited 0. It has not been possible	**I have used a computer or a pad** 4. Daily or almost daily 3. 2-4 times a week 2. About once a week 1. Less than once a week 0. Not at all
8	**I have wanted to help or support people close to me or other people** 4. Very strongly 3. Fairly strongly 2. To some extent 1. Only a little 0. Not at all	**I have or would have been able to help or support people close to me or other people** 4. Yes, without any difficulty 3. Yes, but with some difficulty 2. Yes, but with a lot of difficulty 1. Not without help from another person 0. Not even with help	**My possibilities to help or support people close to me or other people** 4. Very good 3. Rather good 2. Moderate 1. Limited 0. It has not been possible	**I have helped or supported people close to me or other people** 4. Daily or almost daily 3. 2-4 times a week 2. About once a week 1. Less than once a week 0. Not at all

In the following questions, we are interested in how much, not how often, you have done the following things

Answer each statement (1-17)

	WILL TO ACT How strongly have you wanted to do the following things **during the past four weeks**?	ABILITY TO ACT Bearing in mind **your state of health and your capacity**, have you or would you have been able to do the following things **during the past four weeks**?	POSSIBILITY TO ACT Thinking about **your life in general**, how have you experienced your possibilities to do the following things **during the past four weeks**?	AMOUNT OF DOING To what extent have you done the following things **during the past four weeks**?
9	**I have wanted to do things to maintain my social relationships** 4. Very strongly 3. Fairly strongly 2. To some extent 1. Only a little 0. Not at all	**I have or would have been able to do things to maintain my social relationships** 4. Yes, without any difficulty 3. Yes, but with some difficulty 2. Yes, but with a lot of difficulty 1. Not without help from another person 0. Not even with help	**My possibilities to do things to maintain my social relationships have been** 4. Very good 3. Rather good 2. Moderate 1. Limited 0. It has not been possible	**I have done things to maintain my social relationships** 4. Very much 3. Quite a lot 2. To some extent 1. Only a little 0. Not at all
10	**I have wanted to take actions to make new acquaintances** 4. Very strongly 3. Fairly strongly 2. To some extent 1. Only a little 0. Not at all	**I have or would have been able to take actions to make new acquaintances** 4. Yes, without any difficulty 3. Yes, but with some difficulty 2. Yes, but with a lot of difficulty 1. Not without help from another person 0. Not even with help	**My possibilities to take actions to make new acquaintances have been** 4. Very good 3. Rather good 2. Moderate 1. Limited 0. It has not been possible	**I have taken actions to make new acquaintances** 4. Very much 3. Quite a lot 2. To some extent 1. Only a little 0. Not at all
11	**I have wanted to take responsibility for furthering matters relating to my own life** 4. Very strongly 3. Fairly strongly 2. To some extent 1. Only a little 0. Not at all	**I have or would have been able to take responsibility for furthering matters relating to my own life** 4. Yes, without any difficulty 3. Yes, but with some difficulty 2. Yes, but with a lot of difficulty 1. Not without help from another person 0. Not even with help	**My possibilities to take responsibility for furthering matters relating to my own life have been** 4. Very good 3. Rather good 2. Moderate 1. Limited 0. It has not been possible	**I have taken responsibility for furthering matters relating to my own life** 4. Very much 3. Quite a lot 2. To some extent 1. Only a little 0. Not at all
12	**I have wanted to take responsibility for promoting societal or public matters** 4. Very strongly 3. Fairly strongly 2. To some extent 1. Only a little 0. Not at all	**I have or would have been able to take responsibility for promoting societal or public matters** 4. Yes, without any difficulty 3. Yes, but with some difficulty 2. Yes, but with a lot of difficulty 1. Not without help from another person 0. Not even with help	**My possibilities to take responsibility for promoting societal or public matters have been** 4. Very good 3. Rather good 2. Moderate 1. Limited 0. It has not been possible	**I have taken responsibility for promoting societal or public matters** 4. Very much 3. Quite a lot 2. To some extent 1. Only a little 0. Not at all

Answer each statement (1-17)

	WILL TO ACT	ABILITY TO ACT	POSSIBILITY TO ACT	AMOUNT OF DOING
	How strongly have you wanted to do the following things **during the past four weeks**?	Bearing in mind **your state of health and your capacity**, have you or would you have been able to do the following things **during the past four weeks**?	Thinking about **your life in general**, how have you experienced your possibilities to do the following things **during the past four weeks**?	To what extent have you done the following things **during the past four weeks**?
13	**I have wanted to do things to make my days more interesting or delightful** 4. Very strongly 3. Fairly strongly 2. To some extent 1. Only a little 0. Not at all	**I have or would have been able to do things to make my days more interesting or delightful** 4. Yes, without any difficulty 3. Yes, but with some difficulty 2. Yes, but with a lot of difficulty 1. Not without help from another person 0. Not even with help	**My possibilities to do things to make my days more interesting or delightful have been** 4. Very good 3. Rather good 2. Moderate 1. Limited 0. It has not been possible	**I have done things to make my days more interesting or delightful** 4. Very much 3. Quite a lot 2. To some extent 1. Only a little 0. Not at all
14	**I have wanted to improve or maintain the coziness of my home** 4. Very strongly 3. Fairly strongly 2. To some extent 1. Only a little 0. Not at all	**I have or would have been able to improve or maintain the coziness of my home** 4. Yes, without any difficulty 3. Yes, but with some difficulty 2. Yes, but with a lot of difficulty 1. Not without help from another person 0. Not even with help	**My possibilities to improve or maintain the coziness of my home have been** 4. Very good 3. Rather good 2. Moderate 1. Limited 0. It has not been possible	**I have improved or maintained the coziness of my home** 4. Very much 3. Quite a lot 2. To some extent 1. Only a little 0. Not at all
15	**I have wanted to take care of my external appearance** 4. Very strongly 3. Fairly strongly 2. To some extent 1. Only a little 0. Not at all	**I have or would have been able to take care of my external appearance** 4. Yes, without any difficulty 3. Yes, but with some difficulty 2. Yes, but with a lot of difficulty 1. Not without help from another person 0. Not even with help	**My possibilities to take care of my external appearance have been** 4. Very good 3. Rather good 2. Moderate 1. Limited 0. It has not been possible	**I have taken care of my external appearance** 4. Very much 3. Quite a lot 2. To some extent 1. Only a little 0. Not at all
16	**I have wanted to ensure that my financial affairs are in order** 4. Very strongly 3. Fairly strongly 2. To some extent 1. Only a little 0. Not at all	**I have or would have been able to ensure that my financial affairs are in order** 4. Yes, without any difficulty 3. Yes, but with some difficulty 2. Yes, but with a lot of difficulty 1. Not without help from another person 0. Not even with help	**My possibilities to ensure that my financial affairs are in order have been** 4. Very good 3. Rather good 2. Moderate 1. Limited 0. It has not been possible	**I have ensured that my financial affairs are in order** 4. Very much 3. Quite a lot 2. To some extent 1. Only a little 0. Not at all
17	**I have wanted to take action to further matters according to my faith or worldview** 4. Very strongly 3. Fairly strongly 2. To some extent 1. Only a little 0. Not at all	**I have or would have been able to take action to further matters according to my faith or worldview** 4. Yes, without any difficulty 3. Yes, but with some difficulty 2. Yes, but with a lot of difficulty 1. Not without help from another person 0. Not even with help	**My possibilities to take action to further matters according to my faith or worldview have been** 4. Very good 3. Rather good 2. Moderate 1. Limited 0. It has not been possible	**I have taken action to further matters according to my faith or worldview** 4. Very much 3. Quite a lot 2. To some extent 1. Only a little 0. Not at all

MIX
Papier aus verantwortungsvollen Quellen
Paper from responsible sources
FSC® C105338
FSC
www.fsc.org

If you have any concerns about our products,
you can contact us on
ProductSafety@springernature.com

In case Publisher is established outside the EU,
the EU authorized representative is:
Springer Nature Customer Service Center GmbH
Europaplatz 3, 69115 Heidelberg, Germany

Printed by Libri Plureos GmbH
in Hamburg, Germany